bikini fit

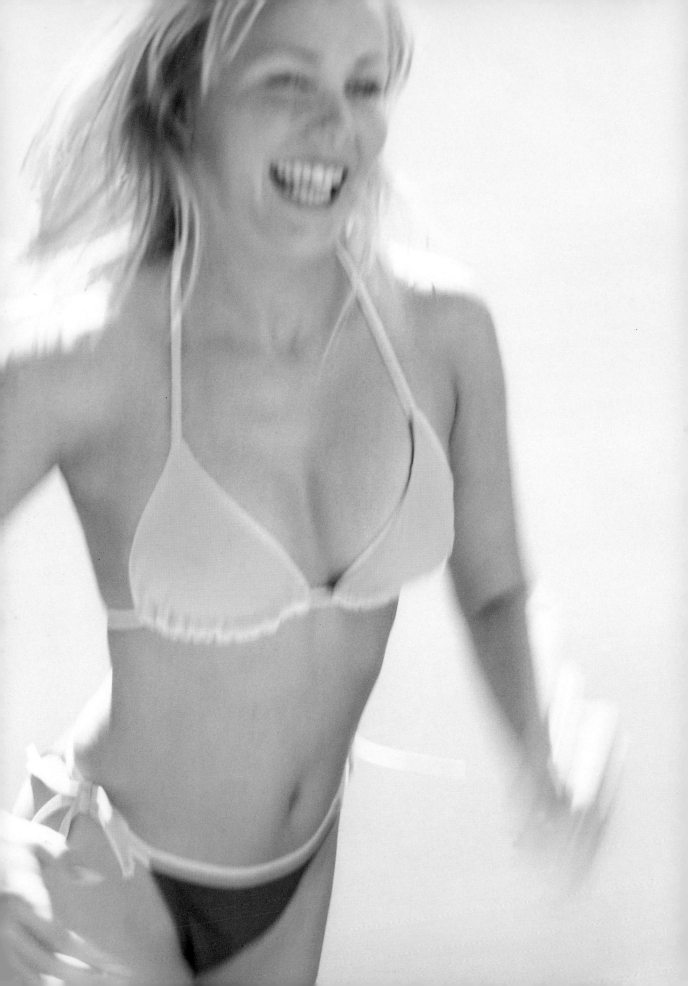

bikini fit

the 4-week plan

Foreword by Chrissie Gallagher-Mundy

Edited by Jo Lethaby

hamlyn

First published in Great Britain in 2003 by
Hamlyn, a division of Octopus Publishing Group Ltd
2–4 Heron Quays, London E14 4JP

Distributed in the United States and Canada by
Sterling Publishing Co., Inc.
387 Park Avenue South, New York, NY 10016-8810

ISBN 0 600 60756 9

A CIP catalogue record for this book is available from
the British Library

Printed and bound in China

10 9 8 7 6 5 4 3 2 1

SAFETY NOTE

While all reasonable care has been taken during the preparation
of this book, neither the publishers, editors, nor the author can
accept responsibility for any consequences arising from the use
of this information. The information it contains is not intended to
take the place of treatment by a qualified medical practitioner.
You are urged to consult a healthcare professional to check
whether an exercise or weight loss plan is right for you before
embarking on it. While the advice and the step-by-step
instructions have been devised to avoid strain, the publisher
cannot accept legal responsibility for any illness or injury
sustained while following the exercises and diet plans.

Some of the material in this book has appeared in *10-Minute
Facelift* (Tessa Thomas), *28-Day Vitality Plan* (Anna Selby),
Fat-Burner Workout (Chrissie Gallagher-Mundy) and *Home
Health Sanctuary* (Anna Selby), also published by Hamlyn.

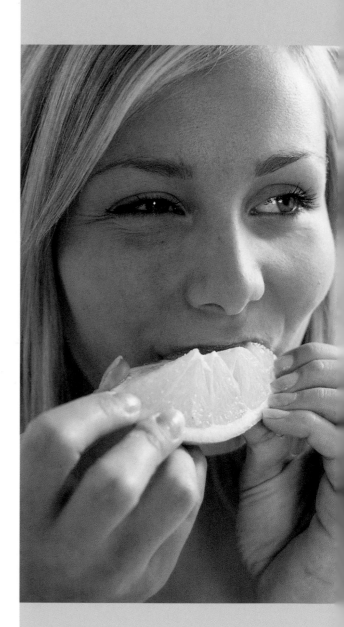

contents

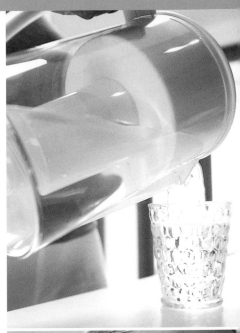

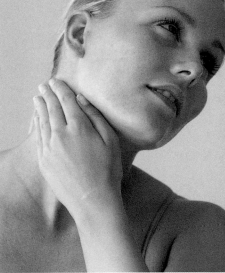

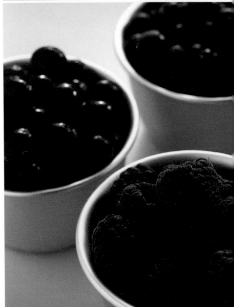

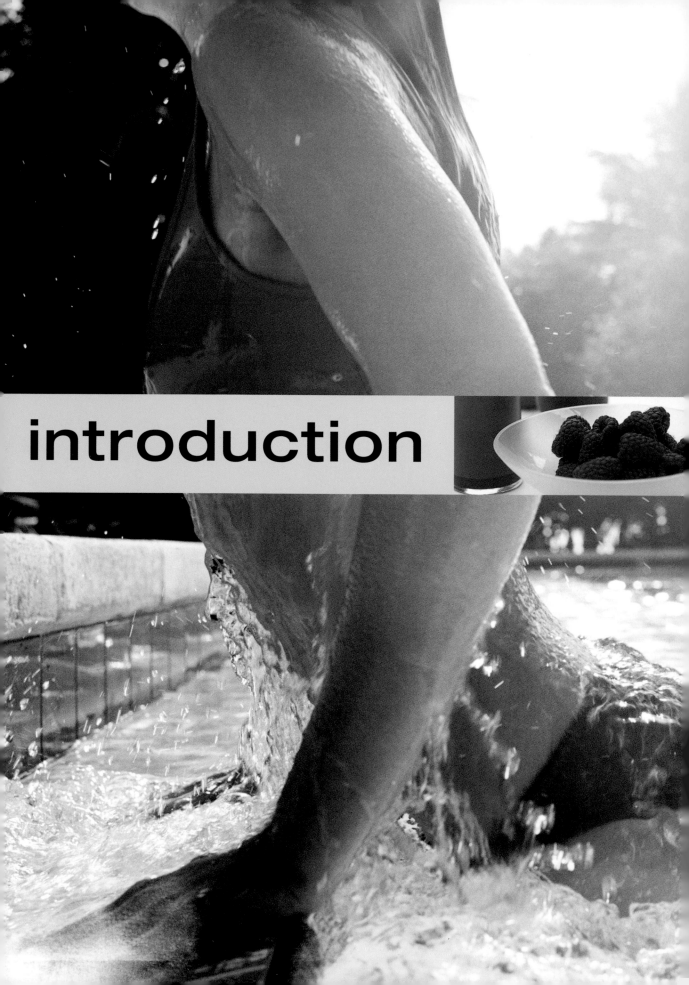

introduction

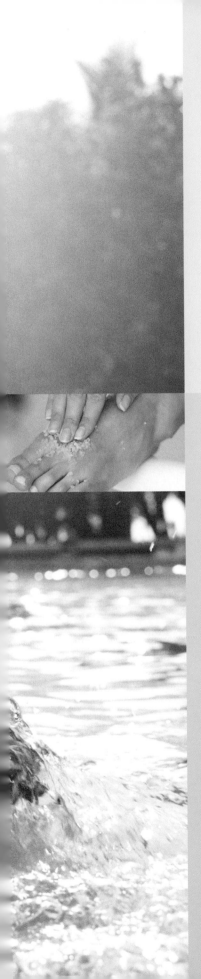

foreword

So you want to get bikini fit? Well this book will take you there!
What does 'bikini fit' mean? It means looking at your body and
face and getting them into tiptop condition. Easy to say, harder
to do, but this book will guide you through the process step by
step – and it needn't take long!

When we come to the end of winter, we start to look towards
spring, but it can be hard to get going when you haven't been
active for so long.

During the winter we tend to cover our bodies with layers of
clothes and forget about how our flesh and muscles look
underneath! So it can be a shock when you realize that you
have to take your clothes off in the hot weather!

But don't despair – this book is here to kick-start your good
spring habits and slough off your winter sloth!

Divided into a four-week plan, it provides dietary, fitness and
beauty advice that will leave you feeling buffed up, full of energy
and confidence. So perfect the plan, pick your outfit and dare to
bare your best on the beach this season!

Chrissie Gallagher-Mundy

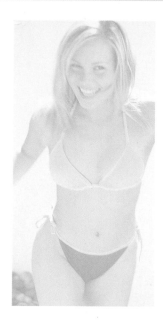

so you want to be bikini fit?

Are you worried how you are going to look in your bikini on holiday? Rest assured that with a little work and by following our month-long bikini-fit programme you can get the look you want within four weeks. You should see a reduction in body fat, feel fitter and look more toned by the end of the programme. In addition, you will have learnt some beauty techniques for giving your body the tiptop treatment it deserves. You will feel full of energy, and be confident about stepping out in your bikini from day one of your holiday – you will be bikini fit!

be realistic

Start by deciding what it is that you want to achieve. This will help you focus on what you have to do to get there. Set yourself realistic goals for becoming bikini fit. Forget about the ideal body types portrayed in books, magazines and on television; decide what is attainable for you. If you are a size 16, for example, you are not realistically going to reduce to a size 10 within four weeks. You could, however, shed a little weight on the run up to your holiday, drop one clothing size, have a firmer, toned body and have a healthy glow about you. Often, wearing a bikini is simply a matter of confidence and, if you *feel* good, you will be happy enough to wear one.

the bikini-fit lifestyle

All the topics covered in *Bikini Fit* are concerned with your body's health and you will soon discover how much these topics overlap. A healthy diet, good intake of water and regular exercise are all paramount for weight loss, the prevention of cellulite, good-looking skin and hair, and your energy levels, for example. Detoxing enhances your energy levels and improves the appearance of your skin, while exfoliation, massage and skin brushing all stimulate your body's circulatory ·

system. Improved circulation enhances skin tone and helps fight cellulite. Essentially, the key to becoming bikini fit is to look after yourself, both inside and out.

confidence is everything

Don't wait for your body shape to change before you improve your image of yourself. So what if your thighs could be slimmer? Be positive about your good parts instead – perhaps you have shapely calves or good shoulders. Remember, most people on the beach are more worried how they look themselves, rather than how you look! Being bikini fit is not the be-all and end-all. What matters is that you are comfortable with yourself. The chances are that you are reading this book because you are not. Follow the advice throughout and by the end of the programme you will be happy with your body and looking forward to showing it off in a new bikini.

choose the right bikini for your shape

Few of us have the perfect figure but you can make the most of your shape by choosing swimwear that shows off your best features and disguises your worst. Many stores now offer 'mix and match' bikini pieces so that you can have a top and bottom in different sizes if necessary and you can choose the style of each that suits you best. Invest in the best, most flattering bikini that you can afford. It is worth paying a little more if it is the one that suits you best. If the bikini makes you feel good, you will be more likely to want to wear it.

• if you are on the large side

A tankini (a vest-like top with a matching bikini bottom) helps disguise body length and can hide as much of your midriff as you want. Swimwear with hidden control panels is perfect for the fuller figure, flattening the tummy, lifting the bottom and supporting the bust. Skirt-style bottoms camouflage large hips, while deep-cut legs help disguise large thighs. Bikini bottoms with string ties at the side can be more flattering than having hips bulging over your bikini bottom. A sarong that matches your bikini will conceal a multitude of sins. Full rather than skimpy bikini bottoms help hold in your tummy. A halterneck top can have a slimming effect if you have broad shoulders.

• if you are on the small side

A tankini adds length to a short torso, as do low-riding bottoms. A bikini style with high-cut legs adds length to short legs. A bandeau top suits a narrow upper body, or you can boost your bust with a bikini top that has gel-filled or padded cups, or removable air-filled pads.

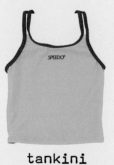

tankini

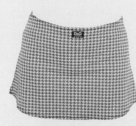

halterneck

bandeau top

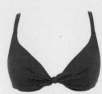

padded cups

deep-cut legs

skirt

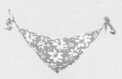

string ties

high-cut legs

how bikini fit are you?

Complete the questionnaire below to assess how much your lifestyle needs to change to get you bikini fit.

1 do you eat breakfast?

a Never ☐
b Only at weekends ☐
c Every day ☐

2 how many portions of fruit, vegetables and salad do you eat each day?

a One or two ☐
b Three or four ☐
c Five or more ☐

3 do you eat high-fat foods (like sausages, pies, burgers, chips, cheese and butter)?

a More than once a day ☐
b Most days ☐
c Once a week or less ☐

4 which of these is your favourite snack?

a A chocolate bar ☐
b A cake or biscuits ☐
c Fresh fruit ☐

5 given the choice, would you prefer to drink?

a A can of fizzy drink such as a cola or something alcoholic ☐
b Tea or coffee ☐
c Water or herbal tea ☐

6 do you have calcium-rich dairy foods, such as milk, cheese, yogurt or crème fraîche?

a Now and then ☐
b Several times a week ☐
c At least once a day ☐

7 how often do you exercise?

a Never ☐
b Once a week ☐
c Most days ☐

8 how much time do you spend sitting in the sun?

a I love sun bathing on holiday and my skin tans easily ☐
b Quite a lot when the weather's good, but I always use a sun creamy ☐
c I cover up, especially in the hottest part of the day ☐

9 when do you wear sunglasses?

a I've got a whole range of fashion sunglasses for every occasion ☐
b I always wear them in the summer ☐
c I wear dark glasses that block out the harmful rays, even in the winter ☐

10 how often do you exfoliate?

a Hardly ever ☐
b Every day ☐
c Every week ☐

how you scored

mostly As

You have a fair bit of work to do to get yourself bikini fit. You are unlikely to be eating a sufficiently varied diet, probably overdosing on fats and sugars and you may be missing out on essential nutrients. Your main priorities should be to increase your fruit and vegetable consumption to five portions a day, eat more starchy carbohydrates such as wholemeal bread and pasta, eat less processed food, and drink a litre of water every day.

Your skin, hair and energy levels are probably suffering as a result of your eating habits but they will soon improve with a healthier diet. Exfoliating all over once a week will benefit your skin's appearance and stimulate your circulation.

You should definitely consider taking up some form of exercise. If you have some excess body fat to lose, try the aerobic exercises in this book for an effective fat-burning workout, or take up an alternative aerobic exercise, such as swimming, at least three times a week. If you are lucky enough not to be overweight despite your unhealthy diet, at least consider doing the toning exercises to firm your body and shape up. Remember always to use a high sun protection factor (SPF) sun cream in the sun and to protect your eyes with sunglasses that provide 100 per cent UV ray protection.

mostly Bs

You are halfway to being bikini fit. Your lifestyle is pretty good but there is room for improvement. You should aim to keep the fat content of your diet down to 30 per cent in calorie terms – if you switch to low-fat dairy foods and spreads, and cut down on processed foods you will get there fairly easily. Try to eat more fruit and vegetables – simple side salads or juices will increase your intake. Opt for water or herbal teas sometimes instead of caffeine-rich drinks.

You would benefit from exercising more – three times a week is the ideal minimum. If you are exfoliating your skin every day, this is too much; you may actually damage your skin in the long run. Reduce this to once a week. In the sun, make sure your sun cream has a high SPF and wear good-quality sunglasses.

mostly Cs

You are already aware of the importance of a healthy lifestyle and are well on the way to being bikini fit. You eat healthily and provide your body with a good variety of nutrients while steering clear of 'empty calories'. Your overall health, vitality and the condition of your skin and hair should be benefiting from this diet. Your body is also in condition because you exercise so often. Depending on the type of exercise you do, you might still benefit from toning up. Don't get too earnest about your lifestyle though. The odd glass of wine or a little sunshine (wearing a high SPF cream, of course) will actually do you good. Keep your water intake up and you should be looking radiant, all ready to jet off on your holiday.

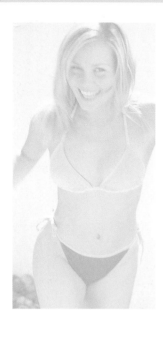

how to get bikini fit

The downside of the many time- and labour-saving inventions designed to make our lives easier is that they encourage us to be less active. In addition, the choice of foods now available means we tend to overeat or eat the wrong things. The end result is that our bodies are often in poorer shape than they should be. If this applies to you and you are worrying how you will look on holiday in your bikini, there are three main areas on which you need to focus – losing weight (see page 14), shaping your figure (see page 16) and beautifying your body (see page 18).

bikini-fit diet plans

The bikini-fit programme entails you looking at what you eat from different perspectives over the next four weeks. The first week kicks off with a detox diet, which helps to cleanse your body by resting it from certain foods and allowing it to process what is already in your system.

Week two advocates a rethink of your eating habits as the best way to lose weight, and the chapter provides plenty of tips and meal ideas to this end. Although you need to continue with this new way of eating generally, week three of the programme places special emphasis on the best foods to eat for your skin and hair, while week four explains how and what to eat to keep your energy levels high.

shape up

Dieting alone does not make you fit nor give you toned muscles. It simply means you end up carrying less body fat. To look and feel fit, as well as slim, you need to combine a healthy, low-calorie diet with fat-burning aerobic exercise and some toning or resistance exercise to build and tone muscle (see page 16). The more workouts you can manage in a week, the quicker you will improve your body shape.

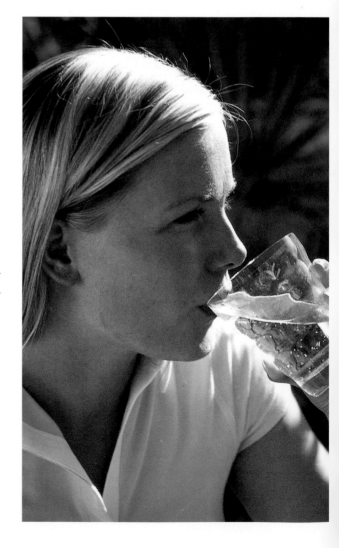

By the end of the four weeks, you will notice a change in the way you look as well as the way you feel.

bikini-body beautiful

There are plenty of beauty treatments you can undertake in order to look bikini fit, but all are best in conjunctuion with a healthy eating plan. Good health on the inside really shines through on the outside in the form of a better complexion, glossy hair and a healthy glow. If you feel good you will look good, and have no qualms at all about wearing a bikini in public.

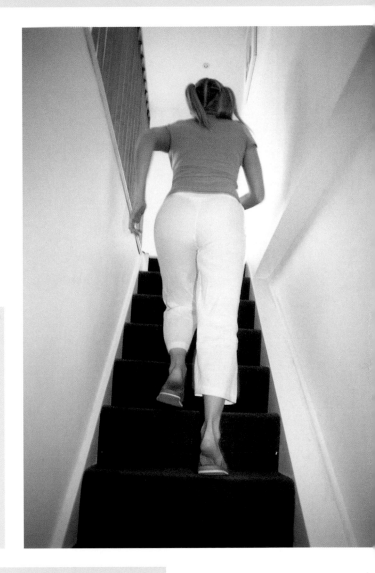

why exercise?

Exercise is not only important for burning fat, it also keeps the body healthy by strengthening the heart, muscles, lungs and other internal systems. In addition, it improves posture, boosts metabolism (see page 16), increases energy levels, improves mental performance and helps combat stress.

be more active

Increasing the amount of exercise or physical activity you do on a weekly basis will help burn calories – even vigorous housework and gardening count. Whenever you go out, take the most active route possible.

• Take the stairs instead of the lift
• Keep walking while an escalator carries you up
• Walk or cycle instead of driving short distances
• Park your car further than necessary from your destination, or get off the bus a stop early
• Do yoga or go swimming in your lunch hour

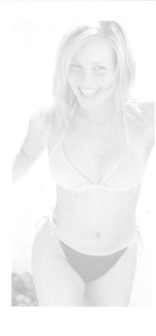

lose weight

Although we commonly talk about 'losing weight', strictly speaking it is actually fat loss that concerns us more. Fad/crash diets may result in a quick loss of weight, but this is usually due simply to loss of fluid, not stored body fat. The effect is temporary and body shape, which is more important and more noticeable – especially where bikinis are concerned – is not affected. In addition, weight lost quickly thanks to an unhealthy diet is unlikely to remain lost. Successful weight loss requires a permanent change of eating habits.

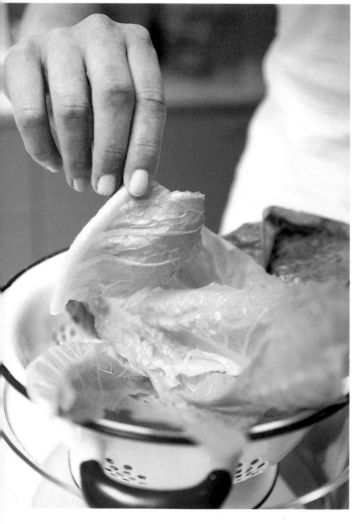

the energy equation

Our body weight is the result of the balance between the amount of energy taken in, usually measured in calories, and the amount used up. This means that if you consume more calories than your body needs and don't use them up through physical activity or exercise, the excess is stored as body fat and you become fatter. If you consume fewer calories than you need, your body will use up stored fat to provide the necessary energy, and you will become slimmer. This process of burning stored fat can be speeded up by increasing the level of physical activity or exercise that you do.

a pound of flesh

To lose weight you need to burn stored calories or reduce calorie intake. Since 500g (1lb) of body fat is equivalent to 3,500 calories, you need to burn calories through physical activity and/or reduce the number of calories you eat for a total of 3,500 in order to lose 500g (1lb) of fat.

calorie counting

The key to losing weight/body fat therefore is to eat less and exercise more. The average woman uses about 2,000 calories daily, so you should be able to lose weight/body fat by eating between 1,200 and 1,500 calories per day. It is fairly easy to work out your average daily calorie intake since most foods now have nutritional information on the label. See page 56 for some calorie-counted meal suggestions and follow the fat-burning exercises throughout the book to burn up calories.

It is important not to become so calorie conscious that you neglect the principles of nutrition (see page 50). It is not only the quantity of calories that matters but also the quality. You cannot, for example, use up your daily calorific total by eating four large chocolate bars instead of nutritionally balanced meals.

A weight loss of about 0.5–1kg (1–2lb) a week is a safe and sensible target. You may lose a little more than this if you have a lot to lose, but the weight loss will slow down as you get slimmer and you will have to exercise more.

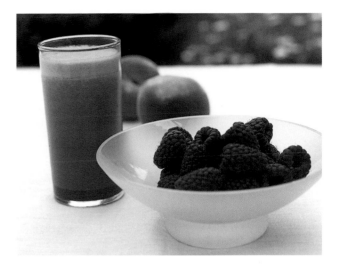

visible results of fat loss

- Smoother skin
- Change in body shape
- Feeling of being less heavy

do you need to lose weight?

The amount of body fat you carry may be more significant than your weight alone. The body mass index (BMI) assesses whether you hold too much body fat in relation to your height. It is calculated as follows:

BMI = weight in kilograms ÷ height in metres squared

or

BMI = (weight in pounds x 700) ÷ height in inches squared

For women, a BMI between 19 and 24 is normal, while the range for men is between 20 and 25. A BMI between 24/25 and 30 is considered overweight. Anyone with a BMI above 30 is considered obese.

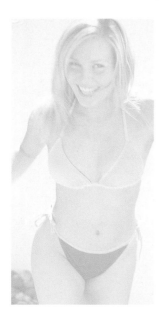

shape your figure

The build-up of body fat usually occurs in adulthood when we are naturally less active than we were as children and when eating tends to be the focus of social occasions. In women, the excess body fat is commonly stored around the thighs and hips, giving rise to the pear-shaped figure. Another typical area where fat accumulates in women is the back of the arms.

Forget fad diets, fancy equipment, potions, pills and creams. There are really only two sensible ways to change your body shape – eat less and exercise more.

what is 'metabolism'?

Metabolism is the continual process in the body of breaking down food, burning calories and creating fuel for the energy our bodies need to function. Metabolic rate refers to the speed at which this happens, and is dependent on factors such as heredity, age, gender, amount of exercise regularly undertaken and muscle-to-body fat ratio. For example, the more muscle you have, the higher your metabolic rate.

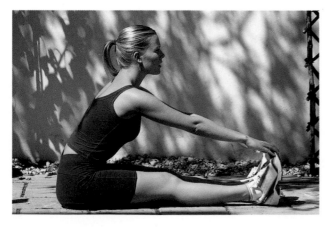

fat-burning workouts

Aerobic exercise involves using your large muscle groups for 20 minutes or longer, which raises your metabolic rate. An increased metabolic rate burns calories faster and so speeds up weight loss. Do such exercise regularly and you will become leaner, with less calories being stored as body fat. In addition, you will build up muscle mass – even more so if you do weight training and toning. Since muscles need lots of fuel (in the form of calories) to function, your resting metabolic rate will be raised, too. The result is that you will look leaner, stronger, shapelier and fitter.

muscle-building and toning exercises

These exercises aim to stretch and tone rather than build up bulky muscles. They aim to firm up specific body areas, although you will not necessarily reduce body fat in these areas. Just as you cannot dictate where fat accumulates in the body, you cannot dictate where it will come off. Fat gets stored all over the body and the fat that went on last will most probably come off first. To shape your figure, you need to attack the fat through a combination of sensible eating and increased aerobic and muscle-strengthening activity.

bikini-fit exercise programmes

A typical exercise session includes:

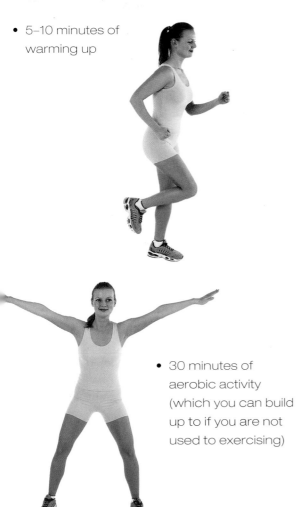

- 5–10 minutes of warming up

- 10–20 minutes of muscle-strengthening exercises

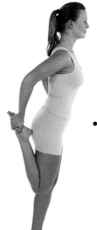

- 30 minutes of aerobic activity (which you can build up to if you are not used to exercising)

- 5–10 minutes of cooling down and stretching out exercises

Each of the four weeks of the bikini-fit programme suggests an exercise programme (see pages 30, 58, 84 and 108), but you might prefer to mix and match different exercises from each week to create a workout that best suits you. It does not matter which ones you choose, but do alternate the different types of exercises so that you use all of your muscles and you don't get bored with your programme.

If you are new to exercising, start out gradually, but aim to build up to at least three sessions (more for optimum fat-burning) of 30–45 minutes of aerobic exercise, and five or six 10-minute body toning sessions each week. If you don't have time to combine aerobic and muscle-strengthening exercises in the same workout, do 'split training', which means that you might do an aerobic workout one session and muscle-strengthening exercises the next time. It is the regularity of your exercise rather than its intensity, which is important. Always remember to warm up and cool down at each exercise session.

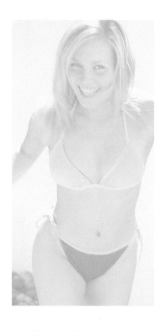

optimize skin and beauty

When it comes to beauty it is natural to concentrate on your face, but you should not neglect the rest of your body, especially if you want to be bikini fit! Caring for your skin is an important part of any beauty routine. Your skin needs attention all year round, not just in summer when you emerge from thick layers of winter clothing and start thinking about wearing skimpier outfits. There are plenty of tips and techniques in the following chapters for you to improve your overall appearance. As always, diet, exercise and lifestyle play a large part.

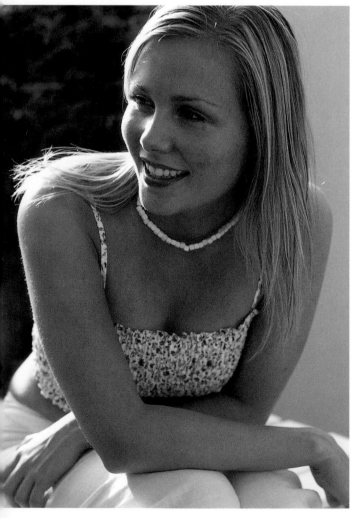

improving your skin

There is no point in shaping up and firming your figure ready to look gorgeous on the beach if your skin and hair are going to let you down. Both suffer from a poor diet and unhealthy lifestyle, so the key to good looks is to become aware of the nutrients you need for glowing skin and shiny hair (see pages 76–81).

home treatments

Exfoliating to remove dead skin cells – once a week for your face, two to three times a week for body skin – is important for overall skin health. It can be achieved using a gentle body scrub (see page 42) or a special exfoliating sponge or body cloth with your favourite shower gel or body wash. The exfoliating action is also beneficial in stimulating blood and lymph flow in cellulite-prone areas. Other treatments that greatly benefit the condition and the appearance of your skin are skin brushing (see page 72), massage (see pages 71 and 97–99) and hydrotherapy (see page 44).

moisturizing

All skin is susceptible to dryness, flaking and blemishes so another key aspect of body skincare is moisturizing. Regular moisturizing helps prevent the skin from depleting its moisture content and protects it from harmful bacteria, harsh weather, the drying effects of some modern fabrics and the dry atmosphere of centrally heated or air-conditioned environments. Your skin's response to moisturizing treatment is accumulative, so the more frequently you moisturize, the better your skin will look and feel. Certainly you want it looking its best for your holiday, when you will be wearing your bikini by day and perhaps off-the-shoulder numbers in the evenings in the cocktail bar or restaurant. You don't want patchy, rough skin – nor do you want sunburnt skin so take care to tan safely (see page 124).

beauty-loving lifestyle

Regular aerobic exercise improves your circulation, which in turn activates and rejuvenates your skin. In addition, sweating when you exercise encourages the production of sebum, which acts as the skin's own natural moisturizer and helps lubricate it. Stress is often a contributory factor when it comes to skin complaints. If you suffer from an unsightly and irritating skin condition, which is curtailing your plans to wear a bikini this summer, think seriously about reducing the stress in your life. Make sure you regularly set aside time for yourself to unwind and ensure you get enough sleep.

combating cellulite

Women of all shapes and sizes have cellulite (see page 70). Many women's Achilles' heel, especially when it comes to beachwear, cellulite can be very resistant to treatment so the best way of dealing with it is to prevent it from forming. Combat cellulite externally with exfoliation, skin brushing (see page 72) and massage (see page 71), which all help break down fatty deposits. It can also be helped from the inside by taking regular exercise (especially walking, swimming and cycling), drinking lots of water, eating plenty of fruit and vegetables and losing weight.

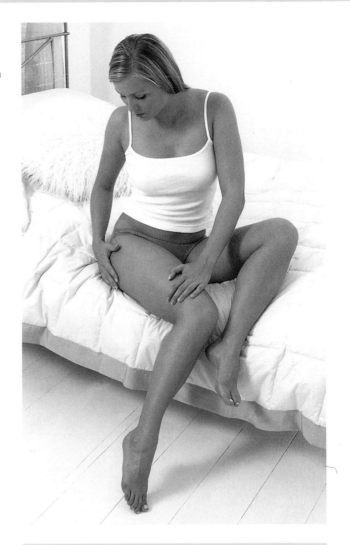

skincare

As well as feeding your skin by eating foods rich in nutrients, total skin care involves using appropriate body and face cleansers, exfoliating regularly to gently slough off dead skin cells and using moisturizers after bathing that contain both hydrating ingredients and antioxidants.

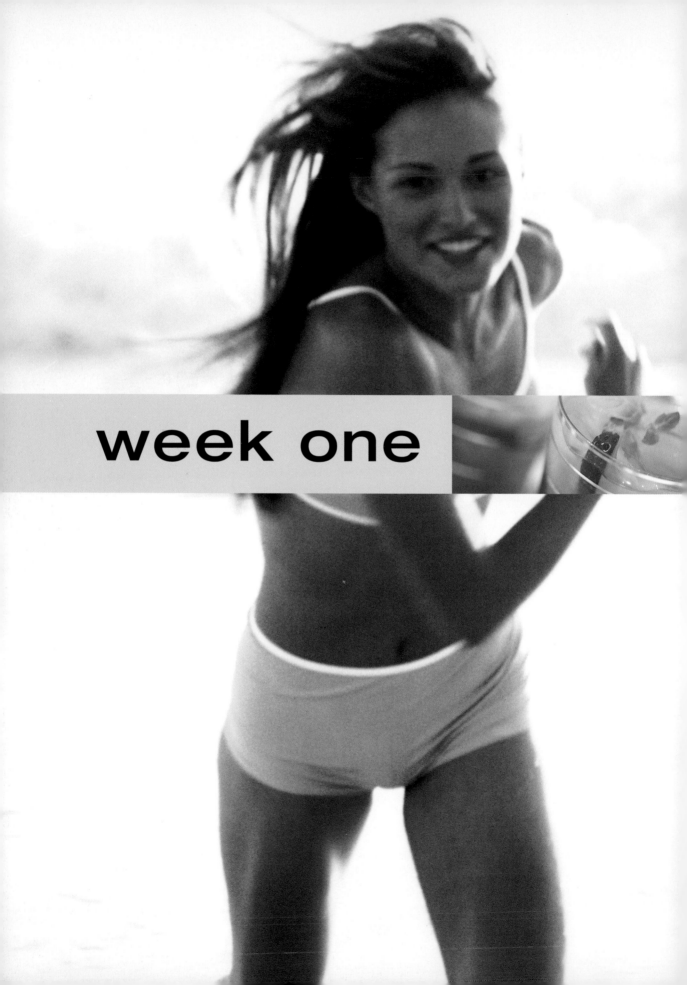

week one

Our bodies face constant assault from pollution, stress and everyday toxins. Over time the effects of toxin build-up can manifest in everything from headaches and digestive problems to cancer and heart disease. Start getting bikini fit by detoxing to give your body a helping hand to cleanse and repair itself, restoring balance to the system.

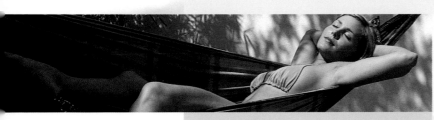

detox

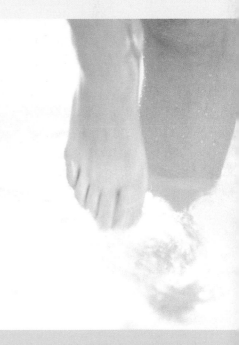

7-stage detox diet •
kickstart your weight loss •
revive energy levels •
invigorate the skin •
gentle exercise •

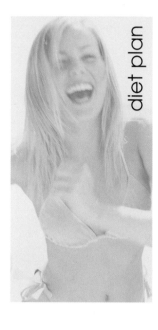

diet plan

why detox?

Not only do many of us overeat through habit, but our food has lost much of its nutritional value through processing and is packed full of fat, sugar and additives. When we pour these and other toxins like alcohol and caffeine into our bodies, our metabolism prioritizes rendering them harmless or 'detoxed'. This leaves less energy for the everyday processes of cleansing, healing and renewal. Over time, the body cannot keep up the pace, strain on the overworked liver and kidneys shows and the body's performance slows down.

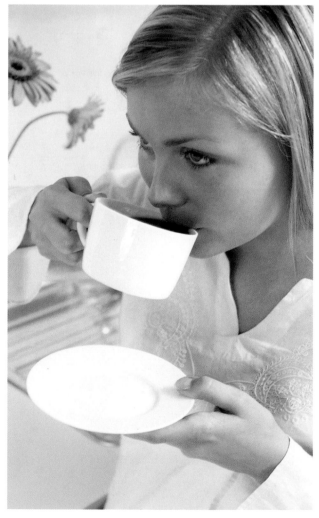

what is a detox diet?

A detoxification diet allows two things to happen. Firstly, by abstaining from certain foods you stop overloading your body with harmful substances and, secondly, you give it plenty of the right nutrients to actually speed up the elimination of old toxins and unwanted waste and promote cell renewal. As the cells are rejuvenated, you become healthier and you look and feel younger!

Since much of the nutritional value of food is lost in its cooking and processing, eating food that is as close to its natural state as possible is at the core of any detox plan. Raw fresh fruit and vegetables, lentils, pulses and wholegrain rice therefore play a large part in a detox diet.

You also have to cut out certain things for the detoxification process to work:

- Smoking
- Alcohol
- Over-the-counter drugs (but check with your doctor about prescribed drugs)
- Caffeine.

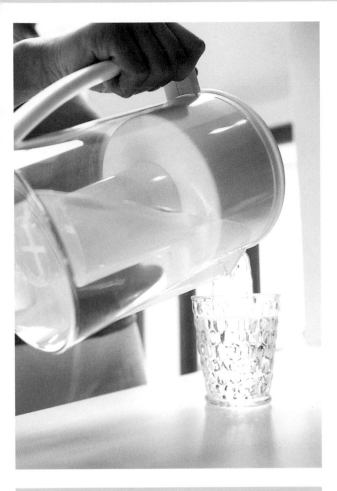

when is it best to detox?

Although the first few days of a detox diet can be an endurance test, within a relatively short time you will feel re-energized and your skin will be glowing. As your body starts to clear itself of trapped toxins, you usually feel tired and may suffer muscle pains, mood swings, headaches and skin problems, but do persevere. Detoxing is actually much easier than you think, but help yourself by choosing the right time to detox.

Since you are probably starting your bikini-fit programme in spring or early summer ready for your summer holiday there should be a good seasonal supply of fresh, locally grown fruit and vegetables and you should feel less need to eat for comfort or warmth. Make sure you are not going to be very busy or stressed or have a particularly social time – with all the temptations of food and drink that go with it! If you work, try and start the detox diet on a Friday so you are not wilting over the office desk during the energy-sapping early days.

detox therapies

By undertaking a detoxifying programme you can help your liver, kidneys and skin, the main organs of detoxification. Detoxification does not involve diet alone. Therapies that help the general detox process by improving the circulation of blood and lymph (the body's internal irrigation system which carries away toxins) include:

- deep breathing exercises
- exfoliation (see page 42)
- hydrotherapy (see page 44)
- massage (see page 71)
- skin brushing (see page 72)
- exercise (which additionally increases the elimination of toxins through the lungs, as air, and through the skin, as sweat).

rehydrating your body

Water is the quickest and purest way of flushing toxins out of your system, and keeping your body in top condition. Since every internal metabolic reaction within our bodies relies on water, the average person needs to take in at least 1.8 litres (3 pints) of water daily (coffee, tea, beer, coke and saccharine-sweetened fizzy drinks do not count) to function optimally – more if you do strenuous activity. Herbal teas and fresh fruit and vegetables, juiced or eaten whole, do count towards water intake because of their high water content.

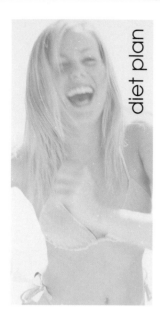

diet plan

7-stage detox diet

Although this detox diet could be adapted to last anything from one to four weeks, one week of detoxing should be sufficient to start your bikini-fit programme. This detox diet is split into seven stages, so in a week-long detox each stage will last one day (in a two-week regime each stage would last two days and so on). It is important to follow the plan in the order given. After the liquids-only stage (Stage 1) you must come back to food slowly or you will overload the digestive system, undo all you have achieved and even feel quite unwell.

the 7 detox stages

Stage 1   Liquids only
Stage 2   Liquid and fruit only
Stage 3   Add raw vegetables
Stage 4   Add cooked vegetables and brown rice
Stage 5   Add beans, lentils, nuts and seeds
Stage 6   Add grains and live yogurt
Stage 7   Add fish

caution

This detox diet is designed for a normal, healthy adult and should not be undertaken without prior consultation with a doctor by anyone who is underweight, on long-term prescription drugs, pregnant or breastfeeding, or who has diabetes, TB, advanced heart disease, kidney dysfunction, any degenerative disease or dietary restrictions.

detox diet

7 days

good for: elimination of unwanted waste and promotion of cell renewal
++ extra fit: extend detox diet for up to 4 weeks

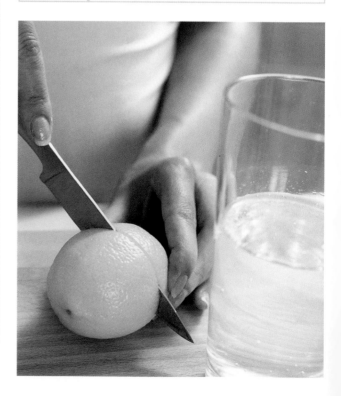

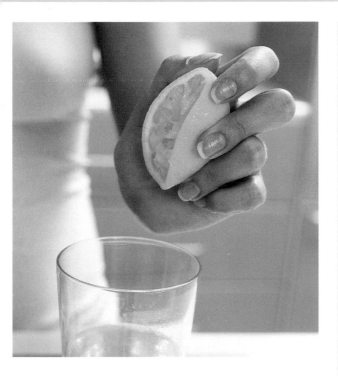

juicing

Freshly made fruit and vegetable juices offer a dose of nutrients unmatched by shop-bought juices. Experiment with whatever fruit and vegetables look freshest. Ignore the froth on a homemade juice – simply give it a stir and drink it straight away as the juice starts to lose its nutritional value immediately.

Peel fruits such as pineapple and bananas that always need peeling. Remove large stones like those in cherries, plums and mangoes, but the smaller pips of melons, apples and grapes can be juiced. If your chosen produce is organic, clean the fruit and vegetables thoroughly and chop them to fit in the juicer. Use virtually the whole item for the maximum nutrients – the leaves, tops and outer skins on vegetables such as celery, beetroot and root vegetables all go in. Juice all the leaves – even the less appetizing outer ones on leafy green vegetables. If the produce is not organic, remove the skins, stems and roots before chopping. Try these delicious combinations:

• **apple and carrot juice** For the best general tonic for cleansing and boosting the immune system, juice together four carrots and two green apples

• **raspberry and peach juice** For a juice that is particularly good if you are overtired or anaemic, juice raspberries [approximately 125g (4oz)] with two peaches. Add an apple or two if you find the juice too thick

stage 1: liquids only

Traditionally, this would be just water – perhaps with a squeeze of fresh lemon to neutralize acidity and stimulate the bowels. However, there are other liquids that have supplementary benefits:

• Freshly made fruit and vegetable juices (see box) can help cleanse and regenerate the entire system. Choose fruits with special detox powers (see Stage 2, overleaf).

• Unsweetened herbal or spice teas such as ginger, dandelion, fennel or yarrow act as useful detoxifiers or circulatory stimulants.

• Broth is another option, made from clean, fresh organic vegetables simmered in water, the liquid strained and the vegetables discarded.

You will not faint or fade away from fasting. You will feel more energetic, not less. Some people, however, should not fast (see caution, opposite), and everyone should check with their doctor before undertaking a detox programme that lasts longer than a week.

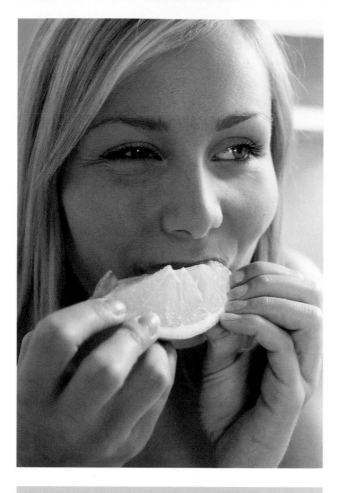

buy organic

When detoxing, use only organic fruit and vegetables if you can or you will be replacing some of the toxins you are eliminating with pesticide residues.

stage 2: liquid and fruit only

Although they often taste acidic, fruits are generally very alkaline foods so they help neutralize the acidic waste that is produced when you begin to detoxify. With their high fibre content, fruits are also good laxatives and will help shift some of the estimated 3–4kg (6½–9lb) of decayed material in the intestines.

• Apples contain a lot of pectin, which helps to remove toxins, and tartaric acid, which aids digestion.

• Pineapple contains the enzyme bromelin, which helps to produce acids that destroy 'bad' bacteria in the gut, encourage the growth of 'good' bacteria important for digestion, and support tissue repair.

• Mango also contains bromelin, and an enzyme called papain, which helps to break down protein wastes.

• Grapes help to counter the production of mucus, which can clog up tissues, and cleanse the liver and kidneys. Their high fructose content also provides instant energy.

• Watermelon is a diuretic, speeding the passage of fluids carrying toxins through the system.

stage 3: add raw vegetables

Include beansprouts – as sprouting increases the nutritional content of seeds five-fold – and raw garlic which is an excellent blood cleanser. Vegetables share many of the properties of fruit, and some of the ones that can be eaten in salads have particular detox powers:

• Fennel helps improve digestion in general and also prevents flatulence.

• Watercress contains beta-carotene and sulphur, both of which are liver tonics.

• Dandelion leaves are a liver and kidney tonic and also act as a diuretic.

• Parsley is a mild diuretic and contains zinc and trace minerals that aid liver function.

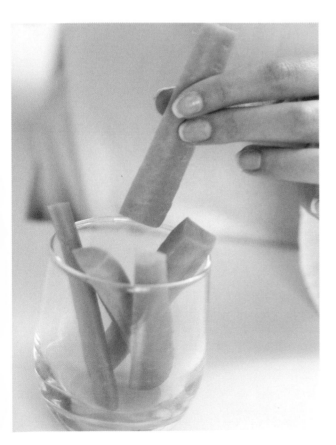

stage 4: add cooked vegetables and brown rice

Cook the vegetables with as little water and for as short a time as possible to retain their maximum nutritious value. Steaming and stir-frying are the best methods.

Cruciferous vegetables (leafy green vegetables) are particularly good for an overtaxed liver. The rice should always be brown short-grain as this is by far the most absorbent type – it soaks up toxins from the gut and is the most easily digested and contains the most fibre.

Among the spices you can cook with are cayenne pepper and ginger, both of which stimulate digestion and encourage the elimination of toxins through the skin.

Vegetables normally eaten cooked that have detox properties include the following:

• Leeks, onions and garlic contain sulphur compounds that adhere to and therefore speed up the elimination of toxic metals.

• Globe artichoke stimulates the liver's production of bile, which speeds up digestion.

• Jerusalem artichoke contains inulin, which aids the growth of beneficial bacteria in the gut. Beware, however, their deserved reputation for flatulence!

• Beetroot is an acidic (as opposed to acid-forming) food, which stimulates the production of enzymes that aid digestion in the stomach.

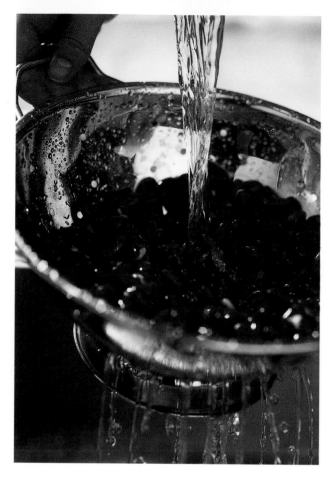

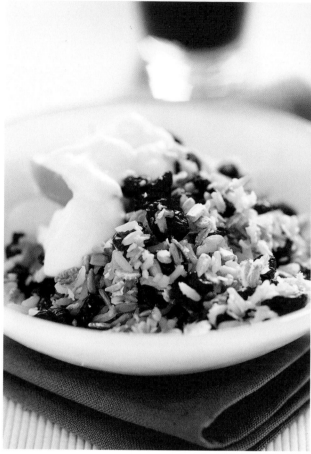

stage 5: add beans, lentils, nuts and seeds

Beans and lentils are a good source of protein but should not be eaten with rice at this stage since mixing starchy carbohydrates and protein can slow digestion. Try to leave four hours between the consumption of the two food types.

Nuts should be eaten raw and unsalted. Like seeds, they provide useful calories in the form of essential fatty acids (EFAs), which are needed by the body but which it cannot manufacture. EFAs also stimulate the flow of bile, which speeds up digestion. Sesame, sunflower and linseeds are all rich sources.

stage 6: add grains and live yogurt

The yogurt should be from goat's or sheep's milk, which is easier to digest than live yogurt from cow's milk but has the same beneficial action on the gut.

The grains should always be wholegrains, which provide fibre to help move wastes through the intestines and trace minerals useful for liver function. Choose from rye, buckwheat, barley or oats – anything but wheat. All help to deliver a slow and steady supply of glucose into the blood (see page 102), enabling the liver to build up a supply of glycogen, which it needs to carry out its detox functions effectively as well as to deliver sugar into the blood for emergency energy.

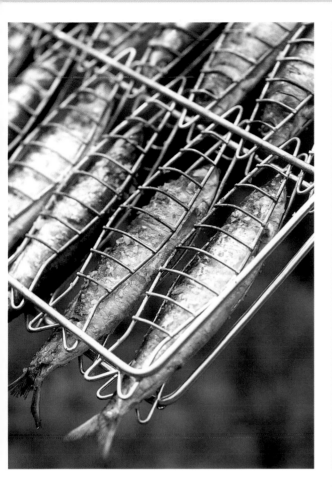

top detox foods

- Apples
- Beetroot
- Brown short-grain rice
- Cayenne pepper
- Dandelion leaves
- Fennel
- Garlic
- Ginger
- Globe artichoke
- Grapes
- Jerusalem artichoke
- Leafy green vegetables
- Leeks
- Mango
- Onions
- Parsley
- Pineapple
- Strawberries
- Watercress
- Watermelon

stage 7: add fish

Any fresh fish will do but your skin will benefit from the EFAs found in oily fish, such as sardines, tuna and salmon. By this stage, you should begin to feel more relaxed and not in a hurry to eat everything you have been missing.

returning to other foods

It is best to re-introduce remaining food types with at least a day between each. By this stage you should be more in tune with your body, which will help you to decide what and when to eat. Add dairy products and meat gradually, as they are high in saturated fats, which slow down digestion. Add wheat last. If you reintroduce these complex foods too quickly, you increase the chances of digestive problems.

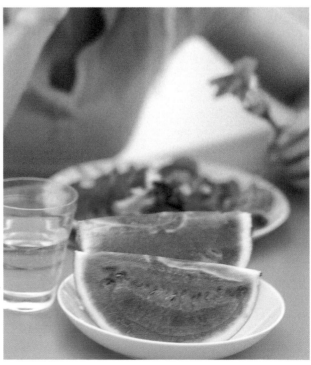

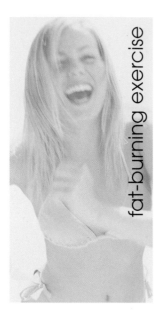

fat-burning exercise

warming up: start of exercise session

Warming up is a must every time that you exercise. It is a way of creating heat in the body. As you move, you build up heat in the muscles, making them more pliable and less prone to tearing or pulling. A warm-up should also involve mobilization of the joints, so that the warmed synovial fluid between the surfaces gives smooth movements. The warm-up phase is also a good time to practise with care any of the moves you might later do at speed.

exercise programme week 1

1 Warm-up (5–10 minutes)
2 Aerobic exercise walking and/or running and/or skipping for at least 15 minutes – see page 32
3 10-minute toners (10 minutes) – see pages 36, 64, 90 or 114
4 Cool-down (5–10 minutes) – see page 34

5–10 mins

good for: preparing body and mind for exercises; warming synovial fluid between the joints, preventing injury
++ extra fit: practise and perfect complicated moves slowly before doing them at speed

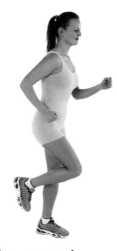

floor march

March for 5 minutes – to music if this helps – until you feel warmth radiating through your body. Swing your arms and lift your knees progressively higher and you should feel your breathing begin to increase.

side bends

Stand with your feet hip-width apart. Reach with one arm down the side of your body towards your knee, letting the body stretch over to this side. Return to upright, being aware of contracting the muscles on the other side of the torso to bring you up. Repeat on the other side. Do 10–12 reaches on each side.

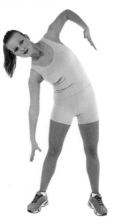

shoulder and head rolls

1 Move your shoulders in several large circles. Lift them towards your ears and 'roll' them back behind you, then move them in the other direction. Drop your head towards the floor.

2 Tilt the head gently upwards to look at the ceiling. Repeat 4 or 5 times. Now look around over your left shoulder as far as you can, keeping your torso facing forwards, then turn to look over your right shoulder. Repeat 4–5 times.

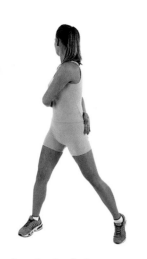

body twist

1 Stand with your legs apart. Swing your arms out and around the body, to one side then the other.

2 Let the movement pull the upper half of the body around with it, so that you start to twist. Let the head and shoulders naturally follow the arms as they pull you around to each side. Do not allow the twist to go below the hips or you may be in danger of twisting your knees. Twist 5–10 times.

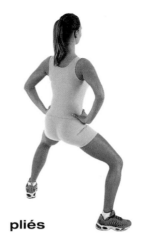

pliés

Stand with your legs more than hip-width apart, your feet slightly turned out, in a wide 'second' position. As you bend your knees, drop your bottom directly between your hips – do not stick it out behind you. Bend your knees – so they align exactly over the toes – until they are at right angles, then slowly straighten again. Repeat 10–12 times.

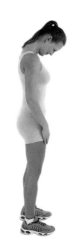

dynamic stretch kicks

Stand with one foot in front of the other with your weight balanced. Swing your back leg forwards, slightly bent, and straighten it into a kick. Perform several kicks quite fast and low to build a rhythm and warmth. Repeat with the other leg.

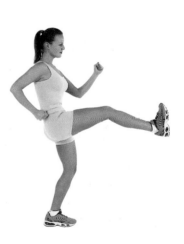

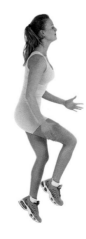

jogging on the spot

Lastly, finish with some light jogging on the spot to get your breathing going, before moving on to your main workout.

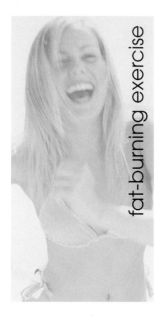

fat-burning exercise

aerobic exercise: walking, running and rope skipping

These aerobic workouts require only plenty of space in which to exercise and a skipping rope. Undertake just one of the activities or do a combination of all three, exercising for just 15 minutes initially and building up to longer periods as you get fitter. Bodies are quick to adapt and with regular exercise you will soon notice a difference. Begin the workout with a good warm-up (see page 30) and finish by stretching (see page 34) to prevent stiffness afterwards.

15 mins

good for: using calories, fat-burning; firming legs and hips; improving overall fitness levels
++ extra fit: increase the aerobic exercise time to 20–30 minutes

walking

Find somewhere you can walk without too much to stop you, like a park or even a shopping centre. Set your watch and keep walking for 15 minutes. When you are walking for fitness you should be breathing fairly heavily. Don't wander as though on a shopping trip, but step out purposefully.

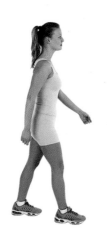 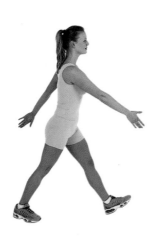 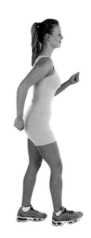

1 Walk for 3 minutes at a comfortable pace.

2 Walk for 3 minutes at a challenging pace with very long strides and arms swinging.

3 Walk for 3 minutes briskly, then walk for 3 minutes with shortened strides (smaller steps than you would normally take). Then walk for 2 minutes fast, followed by 1 minute at a comfortable pace.

rope skipping

Skipping is hard, calorie-burning work, so take it steady and practise to keep the pace going at a reasonable level for at least 15 minutes. The key to consistent rope skipping is to keep your knees bent at all times and lift the feet only very slightly using your hamstrings. Don't move your arms too much either – try flicking the skipping rope from your wrists.

running

Choose your pace – comfortable, brisk or fast – according to your fitness level and keep moving for 15 minutes. Run slowly to begin with so that you can keep going. Place your heels down first and roll through the foot. Breathe evenly, trying to get into a rhythm.

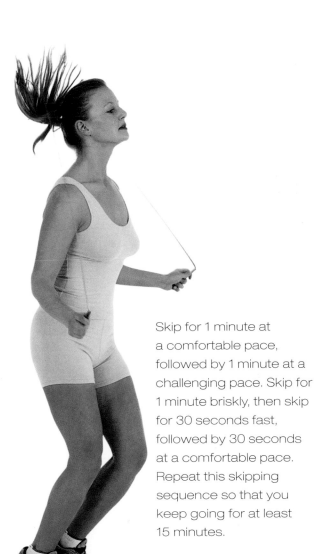

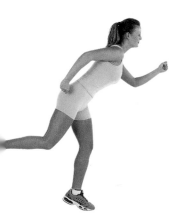

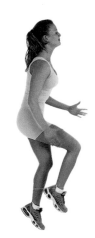

1 Set your watch, leave the house and jog for 7½ minutes. Turn and jog back the way you came. Vary your running strides as you jog – run faster with longer strides for 20 paces then jog normally again.

2 Pick your knees u towards your che and jog 'vertically' for 20 paces then jog normally again.

Skip for 1 minute at a comfortable pace, followed by 1 minute at a challenging pace. Skip for 1 minute briskly, then skip for 30 seconds fast, followed by 30 seconds at a comfortable pace. Repeat this skipping sequence so that you keep going for at least 15 minutes.

variations

Walk or skip backwards, or raise your knees to your chest as you walk or skip.

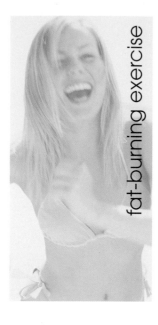

fat-burning exercise

cooling down

After any workout you must give your body time to cool down before you stop moving completely. March on the spot or simply keep walking or stepping gently before you sit down. Once you feel the heat start to leave your body slightly, do the following exercises to stretch the muscles you have used. Stretching returns the contracted muscles to their original length, and helps prevent stiffness and promote flexibility. These stretches can also be done briefly before a workout.

5–10 mins

good for: allowing heart rate to recover gradually; returning muscles to pre-exercise state; preventing stiffness after exercise

caution

The reason for cooling down is that you should never stop vigorous exercise suddenly as the blood is pumping strongly and could cause a blockage. The circulation needs time to return to a more normal pace, so always bring your heart rate down gradually with slower exercise before you stop moving completely.

Cooling down also helps release the muscles from their strong contractions and disperse the lactic acid that accumulate during exercise and which causes muscle stiffness and soreness.

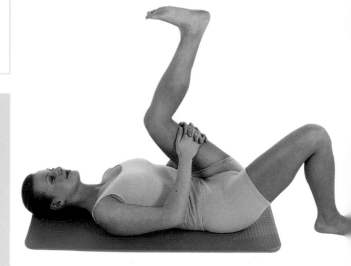

hamstring stretch

Start by stretching out your leg muscles. Lie on the floor and lift one leg up till you can catch hold of it with your hands. Hold the leg as straight as you can bear it. Gently rotate your ankle first one way and then the other. Then gently pull in the leg a little further if you can. Hold and release. Repeat with the other leg.

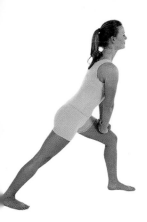

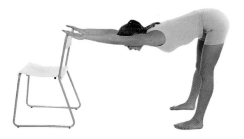

all-over lean

Hold the back of a sturdy chair and walk your legs away until your body is at right angles. Try to relax into and hold this position for 10–12 seconds, keeping the abdominal muscles working for some support. You will feel a stretch in the shoulders and the backs of your legs, and you should feel a pleasant flexing of the lower back (the lumbar spine area). Walk yourself back to standing.

calf stretch

Stand in a lunge position with one leg stretched behind. Bend the front knee to lean forwards, while pressing the back heel down. Hold this position for 10–12 seconds so that you can feel a stretch in the back of the lower leg (the calf muscle). This muscle is prone to cramp, so stretch it regularly. Change legs and repeat.

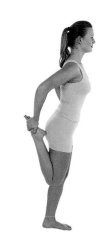

quad stretch

Stand on one leg with a hand on the wall or a chair back to balance you. Grasp the other foot with the other hand. Press the heel of the foot towards your bottom, while pressing your hips forwards and pulling in on your abdominals. Hold for 10–12 seconds to stretch the front of the thigh (the quadriceps muscle). Repeat on the other leg.

swing out

Well done! You have completed your work-out and stretched out your body. Breathing deeply, gently swing and shake your arms around the body, up above your head and down towards your feet – bending your knees.

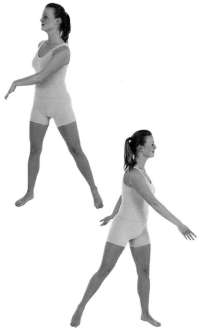

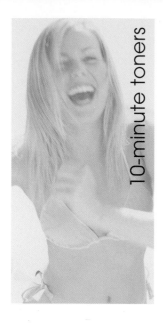

10-minute toners

10-minute stomach toners

The stomach muscles are often some of the weakest in women's bodies, and we tend to make up for this fact by letting our backs take the strain. By strengthening your abdominal muscles, you take pressure off your back and get a flat tummy in the process. Stop if your abdominals start to bulge or quiver at any time during these exercises: this indicates you are attempting something that is as yet beyond them!

10 mins

good for: flattening stomach; strengthening abdominal mucles; improving posture
++ extra fit: build up more repetitions of roll-ups, rope climbing, crossed fists and scissors as your stomach muscles become stronger

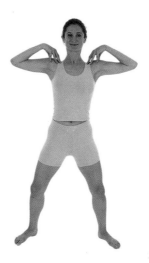

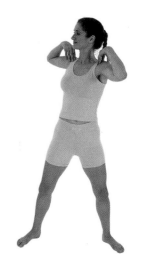

torso twists

With these twists, it is important to remember that it is only the waist and upper body that turn – the hips stay absolutely still and facing the front.

1 Stand with your feet hip-width apart, feet slightly turned out and knees bent. Rest your hands lightly on your shoulders, elbows pointing straight out. Feel your back straight and your tailbone dropping down towards the floor.

2 Turn from the waist to look over your left shoulder. Do 16 turns and then repeat to the right.

upper body circles

This is a more complex version of the Torso Twists exercise.

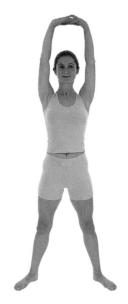

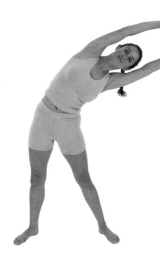

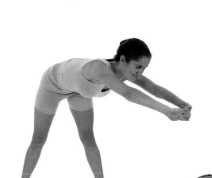

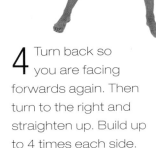

1 Stand with your feet hip-width apart and slightly turned out, your arms raised, shoulders down and hands clasped.

2 Drop down to the left until your arms are parallel to the floor, feeling the stretch all the way up the right side of your body.

3 Now turn so that you are looking down at the floor, but keep your body on the same level. This calls for a lot of work from the abdominals.

4 Turn back so you are facing forwards again. Then turn to the right and straighten up. Build up to 4 times each side.

posture

Standing properly, with your shoulders back, chest out and tummy in improves your shape and makes you look slimmer straight away. In addition, strengthening your abdominal and lower back muscles will make you stand up straighter.

roll-ups

This is a series of exercises that builds up in difficulty, so start with the first one and only go on to the later ones as your muscles strengthen. How quickly you progress will depend on your initial level of fitness.

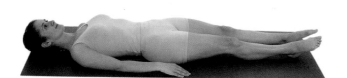

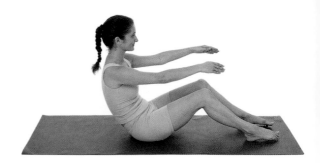

1 Lie on the floor with your legs stretched out and your arms at your sides. Pull your abdominals back into the floor, tightening your buttock muscles under you at the same time. This will cause your knees to bend slightly and your pelvis to tilt. Repeat 4 times.

2 In the second stage, repeat the pelvic tilt, this time moving your upper body off the floor, arms outstretched and parallel to the floor. Your head should come up last. Do not raise yourself far enough off the floor to make your stomach bulge or your shoulders tense. Repeat 4 times.

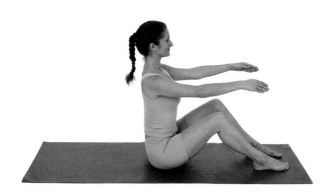

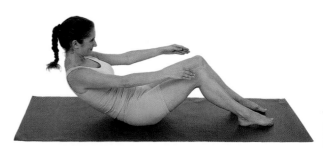

3 In the third stage, begin as before and continue to raise your upper body until you are sitting straight up, arms stretched out in front, head and neck in a long line with your spine.

4 Now drop your head forwards on to your chest and roll back down through the spine, holding on tight to the abdominals. Try to feel your back go down, vertebra by vertebra, lengthening out on the floor. Repeat 4 times.

rope climbing

This is quite a tough exercise for the abdominal muscles, so don't try it until you can do the previous stomach exercises comfortably.

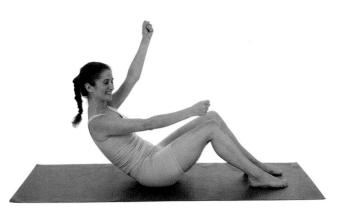

Start by lying on your back on the floor. Contract your abdominals so that you start to roll up until you are about halfway to a sitting position, knees bent, arms outstretched in front of you. Clench your fists loosely, then raise one arm above your head. Lower this arm again and, as you do so, raise the other one. This movement looks as if you are pulling on a rope. If the abdominals start to bulge out or quiver, stop. Repeat 8 times.

scissors

Another tough one for the abdominals! If you are not ready for this, the small of your back will come off the floor – in which case, stop. Remember, the lower your legs, the harder the exercise.

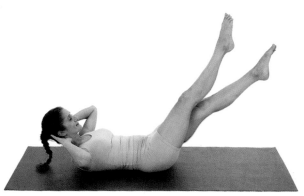

Lie flat on the floor, arms by your sides. Then bend your knees into your chest and stretch your legs upwards. Bend your elbows to rest your fingers just behind your ears. Lift your head and shoulders off the ground and look up at your legs. Pull your stomach well in (raise your legs higher if the exertion is too great). Now scissor your legs, crossing them at the ankles. Repeat 16 times.

crossed fists

A continuation of the Rope Climbing exercise, this is another very tough one!

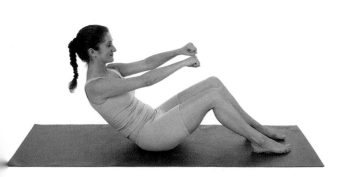

Start by lying on your back on the floor. Contract your abdominals so that you start to roll up until you are about halfway to a sitting position, knees bent, arms outstretched in front of you. With your hands in loose fists, cross and recross one above the other, raising your arms at the same time until they are reaching straight upwards. Make sure you don't tense your neck or shoulders as you do this. When you reach the top, reverse and come down in 4 crosses. Repeat the whole sequence 4 times up and down.

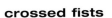

double leg stretch

This stomach strengthener is a Pilates-based sequence and an excellent all-round toning exercise.

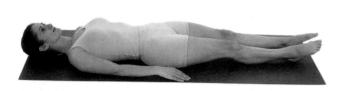

1 Lie on your back on the floor, legs outstretched and arms by your sides.

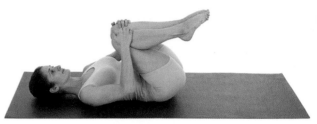

2 Raise your knees to your chest and rest your hands on your knees.

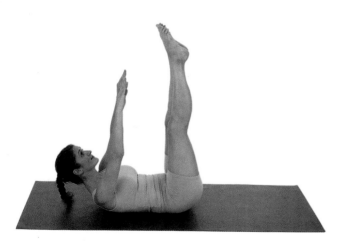

3 Keeping your stomach firmly held in, curve up your head and shoulders towards your knees, but without tensing your shoulders or neck. Keeping the same curve in your back, pull your navel into your spine and extend your arms and legs so they are both pointing straight upwards.

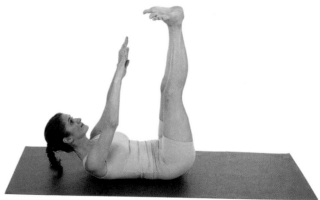

4 In this position, turn out your legs from the hips and flex your feet (the more you flex, the better the exercise is for the thighs).

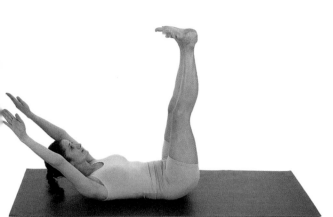

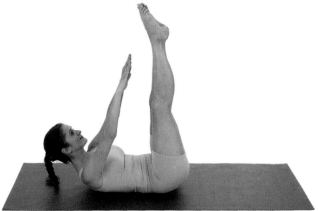

5 Keeping the feet and legs as they are, take both arms back towards your ears and up over your head, then take an arm out to each side in the widest circle you can back to their previous position, stretching upwards.

6 When they are back to their stretching upwards position, point your toes and really stretch both arms and legs upwards. Bring your knees down to your chest and roll your back and head down to the floor. Work up to repeating this exercise 10 times.

variation

When you are lying on your back, the lower your legs are towards the floor the more strain you will be putting on your stomach. Lift them higher and the exercise will instantly become easier.

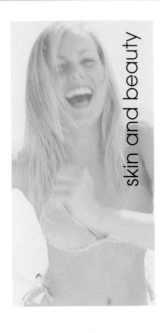

skin and beauty

skin detox

Giving your skin a thorough clean out helps to balance moisture, clean the pores and get rid of dead skin cells, paving the way for a smooth new skin surface. External methods for cleansing the skin are exfoliating (see below) and skin brushing (see page 72), which boost circulation, stimulate the elimination of toxins through the lymphatic system and speed skin cell renewal. Alternatively, the 'inside-out' method involves boosting circulation and sweating from the inside by heating the body in a sauna or steam room or by undergoing hydrotherapy (see page 44).

why exfoliate?

- Stimulates the circulation for all-over body glow
- Encourages elimination of toxins
- Helps break up/prevent cellulite
- Sloughs away dead skin cells
- Clears the pores to prevent spots and blemishes
- Promotes a new, smooth skin surface

rock salt detox scrub

20 mins

good for: complete skin refreshing
frequency: repeat once or twice a week

Exfoliation is a mechanical way of removing dead skin cells. Salt is one of the most effective and simplest of exfoliants. Mix a handful of coarse rock salt flakes to a paste with two tablespoons of olive or sesame oil. Add one drop only of rose or lavender essential oil, if liked. Make sure that the bathroom is warm and that you have plenty of warm towels to hand for afterwards.

Before you start your body scrub, exfoliate your face and neck if you wish using fine salt (rock salt is too coarse for the delicate skin of the face) mixed with olive or sesame oil. Even if you have oily facial skin you need to use the oil as it makes the scrub easier to apply and nourishes the skin.

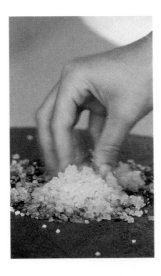

1 Stand under a warm shower for 1–2 minutes and make sure your whole body is wet. Step out from under the water, scoop some of the scrub mixture into your hand and, starting from your feet, massage it well into your skin, using circular movements with your whole hand. Make sure you scrub the soles of your feet, too.

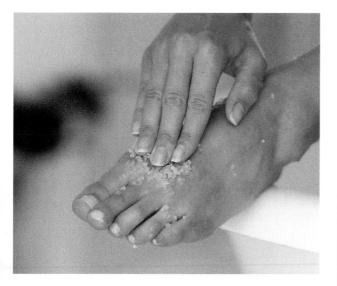

2 Gradually move up your legs, using circular movements all the way. Pay particular attention to your thighs and buttocks as this will help boost circulation and prevent cellulite. Reach as much of your back as you can and then very gently massage your abdomen and chest. Finally, scrub your shoulders, arms and hands.

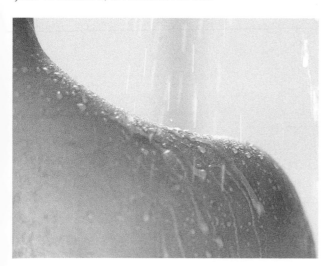

3 Step back under the shower and massage the scrub into your skin under the water until it has all been washed off. Turn the water temperature down to cold and stay under the spray for a further minute, making sure that the water covers your whole body. Wrap up in a warm towel and dry yourself vigorously. Put on a warm dressing gown and lie down for 5 minutes. You should now feel a tingle all over your body and feel completely re-energized.

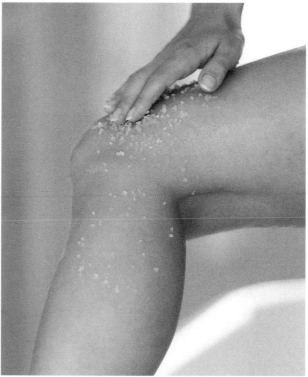

exfoliate for the bikini-fit look

Smooth skin goes hand in hand with a glowing tan. For a lasting tanned look, whether a true tan or from a bottle, you should exfoliate before applying fake tan lotion or sun cream. Shaving is a form of exfoliation as it removes dead skin cells.

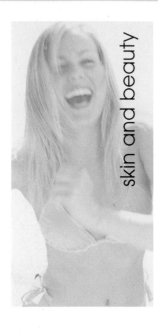

skin and beauty

hydrotherapy

Hydrotherapy encompasses various treatments using water, including saunas and steam baths as well as others that you can undertake at home. The effect of all hydrotherapy is to deep-cleanse the skin and jumpstart the system, stimulating the circulation of the blood and lymph. This is often achieved by extremes of temperature. The ideal way of taking a sauna, for example, is in short bursts interspersed with a cold shower or a swim. In the long term, hydrotherapy strengthens your immune system so you are less susceptible to every passing infection.

15–20 mins

good for: deep-cleansing the skin; stimulating circulation; improving immunity
frequency: do at least one treatment once a week

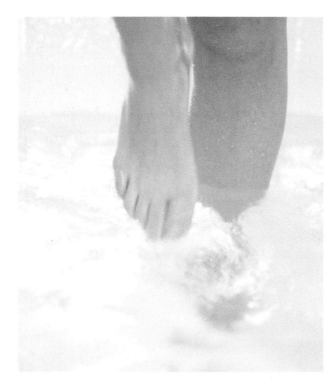

hydrotherapy shower

Begin by showering for 2 minutes in warm to hot water, turning so your whole body is covered in the water. Turn the tap to cold and, again, turn your body under the shower so it covers you for 30 seconds. (Try not to hold your breath, which will interfere with your body's adaptation to the cold!) Turn the water back to hot for another 2 minutes, then to cold for a further 30 seconds. Repeat the whole process once more, finishing with cold water. Lifting your head so that the cold water pours on to your face is very beneficial for your complexion.

Pat yourself dry and put on a warm dressing gown. Sit or lie down for at least 10 minutes. You will find your whole body tingling with vitality – and your energy store will be increased throughout the day.

sitz bath

This treatment works on the same principle as the hot and cold hydrotherapy shower but here you are sitting in water instead. You need two large basins. Fill one basin with very cold water – add ice cubes if necessary – and fill the other basin with hot water, but not so hot that you scald yourself.

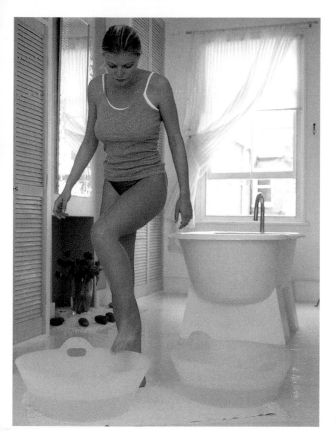

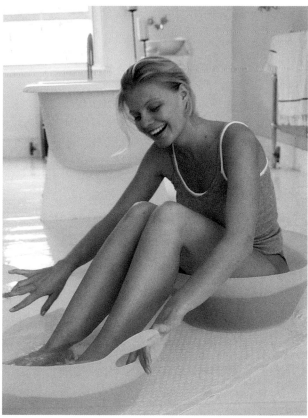

Wearing a short top to keep your upper body warm, start with your bottom in the hot water and place your feet in the cold. This will be quite a shock to the system at first, but after a minute or so, you will start to feel quite comfortable. After 5 minutes, change over so that your bottom is in the cold water and your feet are in the hot. Dry yourself, wrap up in a dressing gown or get into bed and rest as before.

water treading

This is less of a shock to the system than the sitz bath as it involves only the feet. Wrap up to keep warm but leave your feet and lower legs bare.

Fill the bath with very cold water. If the bath is slippery, put a rubber mat on the bottom. Step into the bath and walk carefully on the spot, lifting your foot out of the water after each step, for 1–2 minutes. Get out of the bath, dry your feet well and put on warm socks. Rest afterwards for at least 10 minutes.

benefits of cold bathing

Having a cold bath has a remarkable effect on the circulation. Within about 3–5 minutes of immersing yourself in a cold bath, your blood circulation increases fourfold and your lymph flow is equally boosted. Apart from widening the arteries, cold bathing also boosts the body's production of white blood cells, destroying circulating toxins, and increases your metabolism so that you burn calories more quickly and feel more energetic.

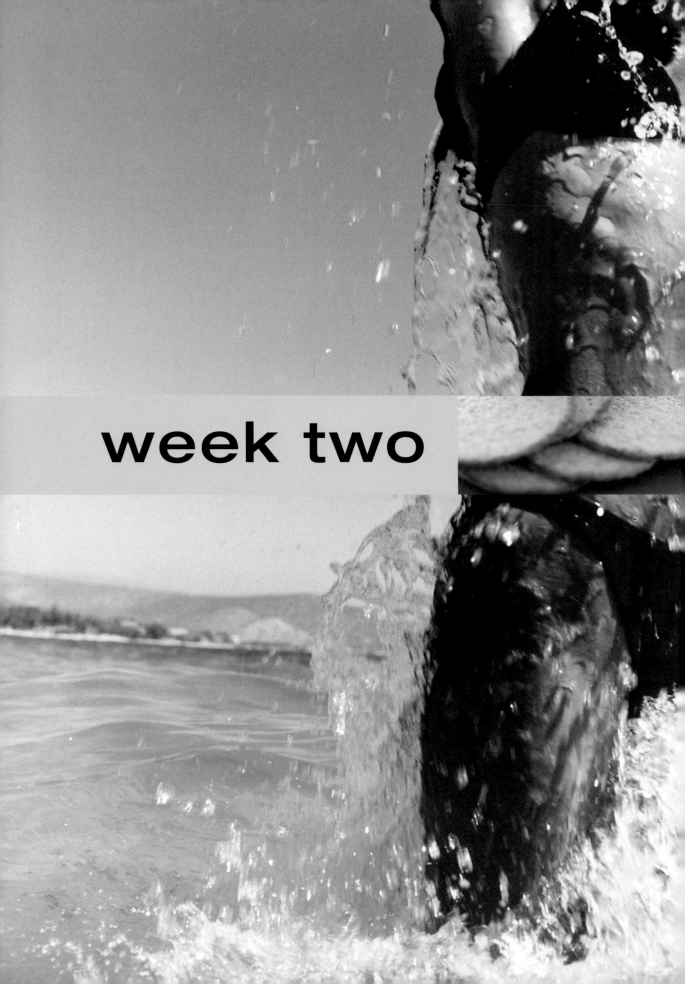

week two

Following your detox week, you should be feeling energized and ready to focus on losing weight through improved diet and exercise. Start by learning to make the right food choices and developing sensible eating habits to keep for life. And make sure you work out at least three times this week.

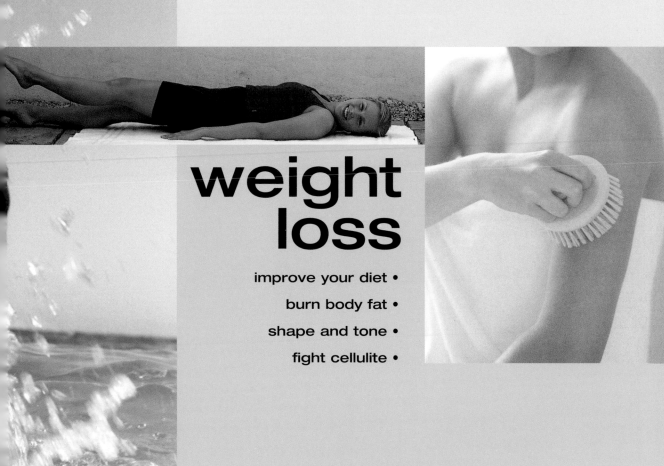

weight loss

improve your diet •

burn body fat •

shape and tone •

fight cellulite •

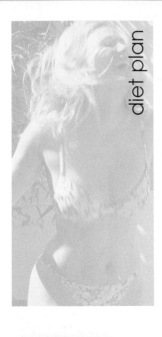

diet plan

first steps

The best way to go about losing weight – and, most importantly, maintaining that weight loss – is to completely revise your eating habits so as to change your basic diet. Don't think of dieting as a temporary project to get you in shape for a specific occasion – something you do short term and then let go to pot. With this attitude you might be able, with any number of faddy diets, to reveal the 'new you' just in time for summer, but once you return to old eating habits you will quickly pile all the weight back on, plus more. Think instead of healthy eating becoming your way of life for good.

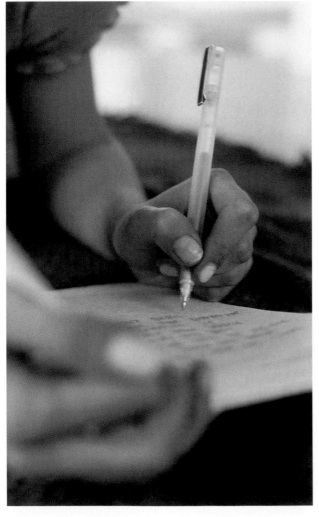

think positive

Having the right attitude is essential for losing weight. Always remember that you are doing this for yourself – no else is going to suffer if you eat too many chocolate bars or cream cakes! It is *you* who wants to be slimmer and more confident on the beach. Make promises to yourself such as 'Every time I am tempted by chocolate I will imagine myself in my bikini'. Write them out and stick them on a kitchen cupboard. This way you cannot ignore them whenever you prepare food or are tempted to snack. Alternatively, stick an unflattering photograph of yourself on the refrigerator door. It will help your resolve no end!

getting started

Clear out your kitchen cupboards and throw out any food that is high in fat or sugar. Stock up with healthy, low-fat low-calorie foods instead – if you have only healthy food in the house you will be less tempted to stray.

keep a food diary

It can be helpful to keep a food diary in which you religiously record all the food and drink that you consume each day. You can use it to keep a tally of your daily intake of calories and chart your progress. It is also a useful record to which you can refer when the weight is not coming off as you had planned – you can check where you are going wrong and make the necessary changes.

avoiding temptation

Try to avoid going food shopping too often to reduce the chance of being tempted by fresh smells from the bakery or fattening foods on display. Certainly, never go food shopping when you are hungry. You could even give the supermarket a miss completely by ordering via the Internet and having your groceries delivered or by getting someone else in the family to do the shopping.

food for thought

It is important not to let food take over all your thoughts when dieting. Having to plan meals, shop for and cook with ingredients you do not usually use means that food can become an obsession. In time, however, these ingredients should become a way of life rather than a novelty, and you can still allow yourself the occasional glass of wine or bar of chocolate as a treat.

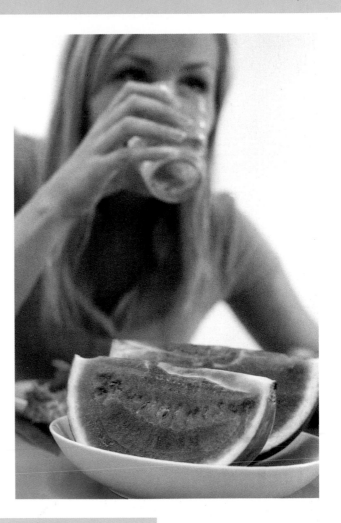

balance your diet

Hundreds of different diets – from special food combining diets to high-protein or carbohydrate-loading – have been proposed as the key to weight loss. Despite all the hype surrounding trendy diets, it is not safe to cut out all fats, nor to follow a regime that excludes all carbohydrates, or one that involves eating only grapes, for example. The human body has evolved utilizing all the nutrients together, and needs each one in the correct amount for our health and wellbeing.

Crash diets that severely restrict your calorie intake are unwise, too. The body's response to a radical cutting back of food is to conserve energy and slow down the metabolism (see page 17) as it prepares for a period of starvation. In effect, the body stores calories instead of burning them.

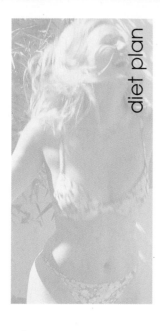

diet plan

perfect portions

To ensure we receive a balance of necessary nutrients, our bodies require the correct quantity of foods from each of the major food groups on a daily basis. For example, when you have a main meal, most of the space on the plate should be taken up by starchy foods and vegetables, with the amount of meat, fish or alternative being quite small in proportion. These principles should still be applied when you are trying to lose weight.

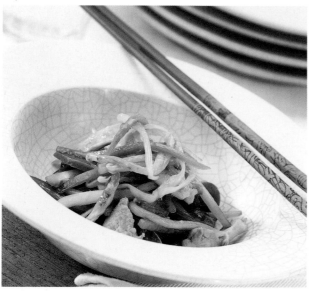

healthy quantities

For a balanced diet aim to have the following daily:
Sugars and fats 1 serving
Protein and dairy foods 2–3 servings
Fruit and vegetables 5 servings
Starchy foods 4–5 servings

sugars and fats

Foods containing sugars and fats (margarine, butter, cooking oils, oil-based salad dressings, ice cream, pastries, confectionery and soft drinks, for example) should be eaten sparingly as they are high in saturated fat or refined carbohydrates like white sugar.

One serving could include a small amount of spreading or cooking fat, and/or a small amount of sugary food. Sugar is best included in a starchy item, such as a cake or biscuit, rather than on its own, so as to limit its effect on your blood sugar levels (see page 102).

protein and dairy foods

Protein comes from both animal and vegetable sources. Try to choose lean cuts of meat and low-fat dairy products to avoid too high an intake of saturated fat. Rest assured that the amount of calcium (required for healthy bones and teeth) in low-fat dairy products is the same as it is in full-fat products. Some nuts are also high in saturated fat.

One serving is equal to:
• 50–75g (2–3oz) meat
• 125–150g (4–5oz) fish
• 1 egg

- 25g (1oz) hard cheese
- 600ml (1 pint) milk or yogurt
- 175–200g (6–7oz) cooked lentils or other pulses

fruit and vegetables

Fruits and vegetables are highly nutritious, providing fibre and some carbohydrates as well as many of the essential vitamins and minerals our bodies require. They are at their best nutritionally if eaten raw or only lightly cooked. We should all be eating at least five portions of fruit and vegetables a day (excluding potatoes).

One serving is equal to:
- 1 medium-sized fresh fruit (apple, orange, peach, banana, pear)
- 2 small fruits (apricot, plum, kiwi fruit)
- 1 slice of large fruit (melon, pineapple, mango)
- 1 handful of berries or very small fruit (grapes, raspberries)
- 1 small bowl canned fruit in fruit juice
- ½ tablespoon dried fruit
- 1 small glass fresh fruit juice
- 1 dessert bowl salad
- about 75g (3oz) fresh or frozen vegetables

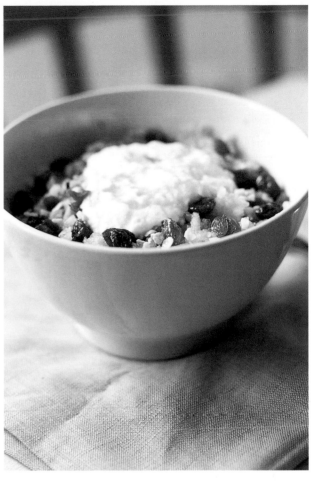

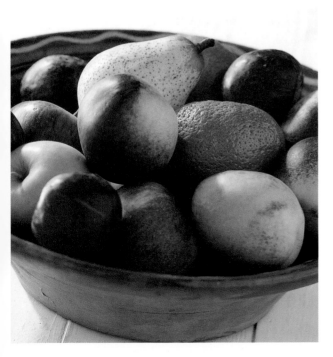

starchy foods

The staple, starchy carbohydrate foods should provide the major source of energy in our diet. These include cereals (wheat, rye, oats, barley, millet), rice and products made from them (such as bread, pasta, noodles, cornmeal and breakfast cereals), as well as potatoes, yams and other starchy vegetables.

One serving is equal to:
- 1 large slice of bread
- 1 medium bowl of pasta or rice
- 1 bowl of breakfast cereal
- 2 medium potatoes or equivalent in yams

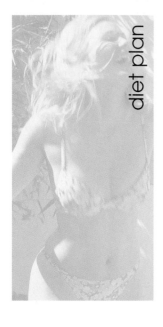

diet plan

low-fat low-cal foods

According to the energy equation (see page 14), we need to consume fewer calories in order to use up stored body fat and slim down, but don't become obsessive about counting calories, especially when shopping. Supermarket shelves are crammed with products that claim to be good for us. Some items, such as low-fat yogurts, are worth buying but other 'diet' versions of foods may be low in fat and/or calories but are likely to be crammed with additives. Avoid buying too much processed food and follow the guidelines given below.

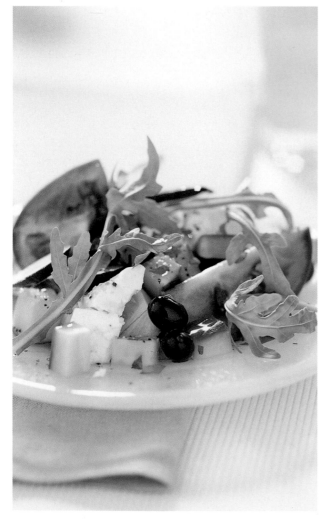

reduce your fat intake

Fat is the most calorific of all nutrients. Cut down on foods that contain a lot of fat (see box, opposite) but don't omit fat from your diet altogether. Simply try to ensure that most of your daily fat intake comes from the good fats (unsaturated fats). Saturated fat, which is found mainly in meat and dairy produce, should make up no more than one-third of your daily fat consumption. To lose weight, stick to foods that contain 3–4g or less of fat per 100g (4oz) serving.

consume fewer sugary foods

Unfortunately, we are genetically predisposed to enjoy the sweet taste of sugar. However, sugar is full of 'empty' calories. This means that it provides energy in the form of calories but very little in the way of other nutrients. Too much sugar upsets your body's blood sugar levels, it causes tooth decay and it is also addictive – the more you have, the more you want. Cut right down on your intake of sugar and sugary foods – be aware that many processed foods are unnecessarily high in sugar and check the nutritional information on labels.

Artificial sweeteners like saccharin and aspartame contain negligible calories and don't affect our teeth.

choose healthy low-calorie foods

Foods that are rich in fibre like wholemeal pasta, wholegrain cereals, brown bread, potatoes and fruit and vegetables are satisfying foods as their fibre is digested slowly so you feel fuller for longer. Low in calories, fruit and vegetables are always a healthy food choice, but avoid eating vegetables served with fattening oily or creamy dressings and sauces, or fruit with sugar and cream. Low-calorie protein foods include fish, seafood, turkey and skinless chicken breast.

shop wisely

Products on supermarket shelves with 'low-fat', 'reduced fat' and 'fat-free' labels attract those of us watching our weight, but what exactly do these terms mean?

• 'Reduced fat' means the product should have 25 per cent less fat than the full-fat equivalent.

• 'Half-fat' means the product should have at least 50 per cent less fat than the full-fat equivalent.

• 'Low-fat' means the product should have less than 5g of fat per 100g (3 ½oz).

• 'Fat-free' means the product should have only a trace – less than 0.15g per 100g (3 ½oz) – of fat.

Be aware that products claiming to be 85 or 90 per cent fat free actually contain 15g or 10g fat respectively per 100g (3 ½oz), which is quite high if you are watching your fat intake.

Another point worth knowing is that some products are labelled with the word 'light' or 'lite'. This is a misleading term and does not necessarily mean that the food is a 'diet' version. It may simply mean that food is lighter in colour or texture than usual. The best way to judge the calorie or fat content of a so-called 'light' type of food is to compare its nutritional label with that of an equivalent 'non-light' product.

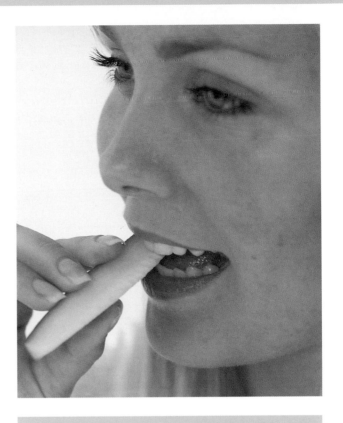

fat facts

The body has no nutritional need for saturated fats, but some unsaturated fat is good for us (especially the essential fatty acids, EFAs, found in fresh nuts and seeds and their oils, leafy green vegetables, seafood and oily fish like sardines, tuna and salmon). However, *all* fats are very concentrated sources of calories (9 calories per 1 gram) and excess consumption causes weight gain.

The average woman should consume no more than 75g (3oz) of fat per day. To cut down on your fat intake, trim all visible fat from meat and poultry, and choose low-fat yogurt, cheese and milk instead of full-fat dairy products. If you are in doubt, start reading labels when you are food shopping.

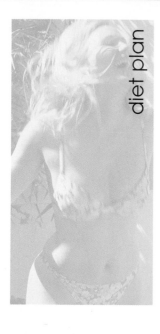

diet plan

lighter living

A weight-loss lifestyle means choosing the healthiest option available. Even if someone else has prepared your meal, you usually have some control over what you eat, maybe refusing second helpings or a dessert. Train yourself to pause before you reach for food – decide whether you are indeed hungry, whether what you are about to eat is nutritional and energizing, or just providing 'empty' calories? In this way you will eventually make better food choices. Thirst is often mistaken for hunger so try drinking water first and then decide whether you are still hungry.

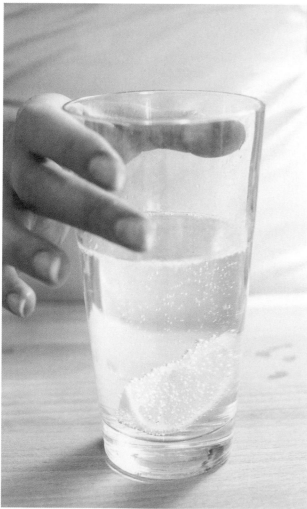

eat little and often

Eating up to six small meals throughout the day, rather than eating two or three large meals is recommended to keep your body fuelled (see page 104). However, you must be disciplined about what you are eating or such so-called 'grazing' could be a disaster.

take time to enjoy your food

Instead of eating on the run, sit down to eat your meal. Concentrate solely on your food instead of eating while watching TV or working at your desk. Eat slowly – it takes 20 minutes for the brain to register that your stomach is full.

drink up

You need to drink about 8 glasses of water per day to stay hydrated (see page 80) – more if you are exercising. A glass or two before a meal will help fill you up so you eat less, but don't drink too much water while you eat as the fluid will dilute the digestive juices and slow down the digestive process. Starting the day with a cup of hot water (ideally with a squeeze of lemon) is very good for waking up both you and your digestive system.

exercise more

Being physically active, especially doing aerobic exercise (see page 16), uses up energy, which will help you burn off pounds faster. If the weight is not coming off despite your efforts, exercise more rather than eat less. Try and fit in extra exercise every day.

keep nutritious snacks handy

Stock the cupboard with healthy snacks such as fruit, vegetable sticks, dried fruit and rice cakes. Keep whatever you find hard to resist – chocolate biscuits, crisps or sweets – out of the house. Your metabolism is at its highest after exercising so if you really must have that chocolate bar then eat it after your workout.

beware of empty calories

Alcohol and sugary foods such as chocolate and biscuits provide 'empty' calories that you will have to use up if you don't want them stored as fat. In addition, alcohol dehydrates the body, can leave you feeling unmotivated and peckish and may weaken your resolve to lose weight.

control your appetite

Learning to say no to yourself and to others is a big part of weight control whether it is refusing a second helping, declining a cream cake at work or resisting the temptation to eat the leftovers as you clear away a meal. Use a smaller plate to stop yourself eating more than you need.

low-fat cooking

Where possible, choose ingredients with a lower fat content. In place of cream in sauces, soups and puddings, for example, use low-fat natural yogurt, low-fat fromage frais or half-fat crème fraîche. Always dry-roast, grill, bake, boil, steam or poach rather than fry food. To reduce your use of cooking oil, cook ingredients like onions in vegetable stock or use spray oil instead. If you stir-fry in a nonstick pan you can omit oil altogether.

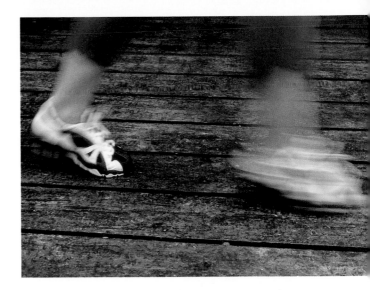

tips for eating out

- Never have more than two courses
- Choose a low-calorie fruit dish as a starter or dessert
- Don't fill up on bread while waiting for your main course to arrive
- Choose tomato-based sauces over creamy or cheesy ones
- Opt for jacket or boiled new potatoes instead of chips or sautéed potatoes
- Be wary of creamy dressings with salads
- Steer clear of dishes that are battered or deep-fried. Opt for chargrilled, baked or steamed foods instead
- Always refuse second helpings
- Opt for sorbets or ice lollies rather than ice cream
- Have a coffee instead of a stodgy pudding
- If you really need a snack at the cinema, popcorn is a better option than nuts or crisps
- To avoid nibbling at parties, have a healthy snack or meal before you go

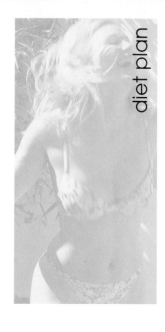

diet plan

calorie-counted cuisine

By calculating your calorie intake it is possible to lose weight, yet still enjoy satisfying meals. Women should consume between 1,250 and 1,500 calories a day to lose weight. An intake of less than 1,000 calories a day will actually hamper weight loss as your body will store rather than burn calories (see page 49). Use the meal, dessert and snack ideas provided below to make up your daily number of calories. Make sure you eat at least five servings of fruit and vegetables daily and follow the other healthy eating guidelines on pages 50–55.

breakfasts

- 200g (7oz) can grapefruit in natural juice (100 cals)
- Banana smoothie made with 1 small banana, 150g (5oz) low-fat natural yogurt, 1 tsp honey and 100ml (3½fl oz) skimmed milk (200 cals)
- 40g (1½oz) porridge oats cooked with water, served with 125ml (4fl oz) skimmed milk and 1 tsp brown sugar or honey (240 cals)
- 50g (2oz) fruit'n'fibre cereal with 125ml (4fl oz) semi-skimmed milk and 1 sliced apple (275 cals)
- 2 medium slices wholemeal bread or 2 toasted crumpets spread with 2 tsps honey or jam (200 cals)
- 1 soft-boiled egg served with 1 medium slice toast with beef extract spread (180 cals)
- Scrambled egg on toast made with 2 eggs, 150ml (¼ pint) semi-skimmed milk, spray oil and 1 medium slice wholemeal toast (350 cals)

don't skip breakfast

Your digestive system needs a kickstart to restart your metabolism after a night's sleep so make sure you eat something for breakfast, even if it is only a banana.

lunches

- Ham salad sandwich made with 2 medium slices wholemeal bread, 1 tbsp low-fat mayonnaise 2 thick slices lean ham and salad (325 cals)
- Homemade vegetable soup with wholemeal bread roll and low-fat spread (250 cals)
- A prepacked 'reduced-fat' or 'healthy option' sandwich (maximum 300 cals)
- Mushroom omelette made with 2 eggs and 5 medium mushrooms, sliced and lightly fried with spray oil, served with salad (250 cals)
- 1 wholemeal pitta bread filled with 100g (4oz) wafer-thin turkey ham slices, salad and 1 tbsp low-fat mayonnaise (300 cals)
- 1 small jacket potato topped with small can baked beans (370 cals)
- 1 soft flour tortilla wrap filled and rolled with shredded lettuce and 100g (3½oz) can tuna in brine, drained and mixed with ½ chopped red onion and 1 tbsp very low-fat yogurt (300 cals)

dinners

- 100g (4oz) diced chicken or turkey, stir-fried with 1 tsp vegetable oil and 1 sliced pepper, 5 medium mushrooms, 1 sliced onion, a good handful of beansprouts, 100g (4oz) courgettes, 1 large carrot and 1 tbsp soy sauce (450 cals)

- Foil-baked 150g (5oz) salmon fillet or 150g (5oz) tuna steak, 5 boiled small new potatoes and 3 heaped tbsp green beans (450 cals)
- Grilled 100g (4oz) sirloin or rump steak, 100g (4oz) low-fat oven chips, 1 grilled large flat mushroom and 2 heaped tbsp cooked frozen peas (485 cals)
- Barbecued or grilled lamb and apricot kebabs, comprising skewers threaded with 100g (4oz) diced lean lamb, 4 baby onions, ¼ red pepper and 2 fresh apricots stoned and quartered on to skewers. Grill or barbecue and serve with 1 tbsp low-fat mayonnaise and a large mixed salad (400 cals)
- 3 grilled extra-lean pork sausages served with a sauce of 1 tbsp wholegrain mustard mixed with 2 tbsp half-fat crème fraîche, scoop of mashed potato and boiled or steamed spinach, cabbage or broccoli (450 cals)
- 75g (3oz) (uncooked weight) dried pasta shells, cooked, mixed with a homemade cooked sauce of 5 tbsp passata, chopped chillies, 2 garlic cloves and 1 chopped onion, and sprinkled with 1 tbsp grated Parmesan cheese (360 cals)
- Homemade vegetable curry and 50g (2oz) (uncooked weight) rice, boiled (430 cals)

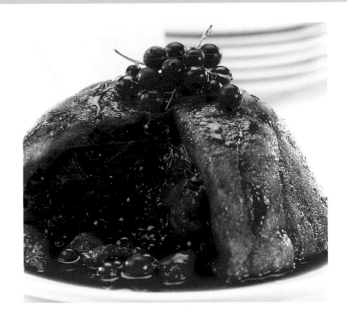

desserts

- 1 meringue nest filled with 1 tbsp low-fat yogurt and 1 sliced kiwi fruit (150 cals)
- 1 baked cooking apple, stuffed with 15g (½oz) walnuts and a small handful of raisins (175 cals)
- 100g (4oz) fresh or frozen strawberries with 150g (5oz) low-fat strawberry yogurt (150 cals)
- 50ml (2fl oz) scoop dairy ice cream or 100ml (3½fl oz) scoop sorbet (100 cals)
- 1 portion fresh fruit salad (200 cals)
- 150g (5oz) fat-free Greek-style yogurt mixed with 1 tsp runny honey (100 cals)
- 1 portion summer pudding with 1 tbsp low-fat fromage frais or low-fat yogurt (275 cals)

snacks

- 2 fresh figs or 1 apple or 1 pear (50 cals)
- 1 toasted crumpet with 1 tsp jam (100 cals)
- 1 medium banana or 1 medium mango (100 cals)
- 1 mini Swiss roll or 2 jaffa cakes (100 cals)
- 1 digestive biscuit (80 cals)
- 50g (2oz) bag exotic dried fruit mix (150 cals)
- 1 tube fruit pastilles (150 cals)
- 50g (2oz) snack pack ready-to-eat apricots or prunes (80 cals)
- 10 black or green olives (75 cals)
- 1 glass wine or 2 small measures spirit or 275ml bottle lager or dry cider (100 cals)

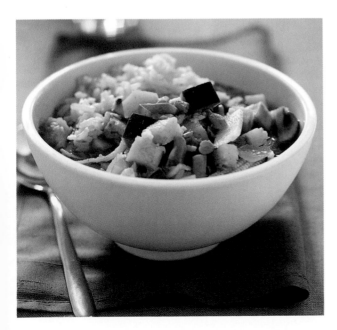

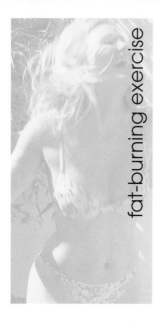

fat-burning exercise

muscle-building workout: heavy weights

Increasing your muscle mass raises your metabolic rate so that you burn more calories, even when resting. You need a 5kg (12lb) dumbbell for this muscle-building workout, which uses all the large muscle groups. When you are comfortable with this session you could try it on another occasion with progressively heavier weights until you can manage only 10 repetitions of each exercise.

exercise programme week 2

1 **Warm-up** (5–10 minutes) – see page 30
2 **Muscle-building workout** heavy weights (20 minutes)
3 **Aerobic exercise** plyometrics (20 minutes) and/or pyramid circuit training (25–30 minutes) – see pages 60 and 62
4 **10-minute toners** (10 minutes) – see pages 36, 64, 90 or 114
5 **Cool-down** (5–10 minutes) – see page 34

20 mins

good for: fat-burning; strengthening and toning stomach and back muscles; raising metabolic rate
++ extra fit: use progressively heavier weights to do only 10 repetitions

technique

Remember to pull in on your abdominals and your pelvic floor muscles when you lift something heavy. As you tighten the abdominals they will support your torso and maintain your posture, keeping the body safely aligned as you lift. Breathe in as you lift, breathe out as you release.

1 March up and down for five minutes, lifting your knees as high as you can while holding a 5kg (12lb) dumbbell in front of you.

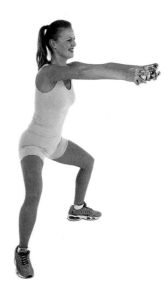

why build muscle?

- If you are trying to lose body fat, then muscle-building is important because the more muscle your body has, the more calories will be needed to maintain it. Therefore instead of your body storing excess calories as fat, it will utilize those calories to maintain your muscle mass.
- Extra muscle will mean you have better posture, you will move with more energy and have an improved, more defined shape.

variation

Use a barbell instead of dumbbells if you prefer. Place the barbell across your shoulders and perform a series of squats (see page 84) or pliés (see page 31).

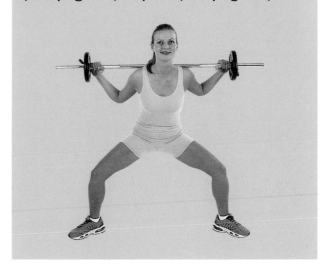

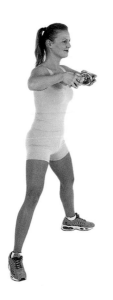

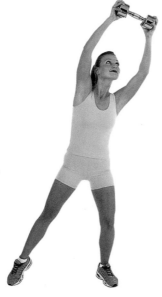

2 Standing with your legs apart, bend and straighten your legs as you press the dumbbell out in front of you and pull it back in again. Repeat this 25 times.

3 Step from side to side on the spot, lifting the dumbbell up and down in front of you. The lift the dumbbell above your head as you reach up first to one side then the other, bending then straightening your knees as you stretch. Do this 25 times.

4 Step from side to side on the spot, lifting the dumbbell up and down, as before, then repeat the whole sequence once more.

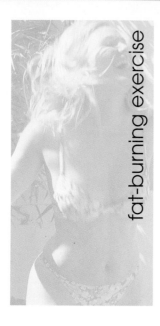

fat-burning exercise

aerobic exercise: plyometrics

Plyometric exercises are high-intensity moves designed to boost calorie burning. Use the park so that you have plenty of room to move. Warm up as described on page 30, then walk briskly or jog for 5 minutes. Jog a length of the park and try one of the following moves on the return leg. Continue in this way for 20 minutes, jogging outbound lengths and trying the various moves below as you come back each time.

20–30 mins

good for: fat-burning; improving overall fitness levels; firming legs and hips

++ extra fit: build up to 30 minutes

bounding

Start by jogging with large paces. As you jog, push off each foot as much as you can so that you are spending longer in the air between each step. The actual pacing will be slower but you will use more energy as you push off the ground.

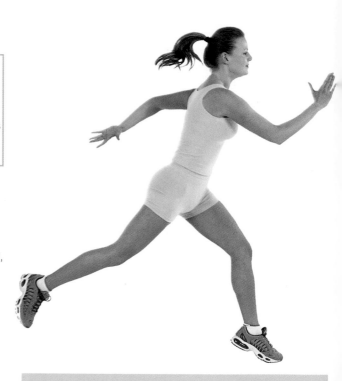

technique

It is important when doing any kind of jump that you check the alignment of your knees. As your knees bend, make sure that your knees are in line with your toes and do not extend beyond them.

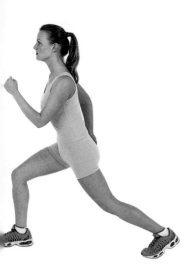

step lunges

Stand on the spot and step forwards into a lunge position. Both legs should be bent, with your weight evenly distributed between them. Push forwards with your back leg to step into another lunge in front. Keep alternating as you step right across the park.

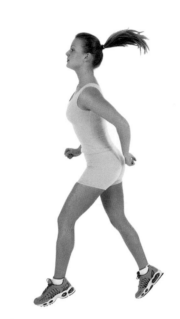

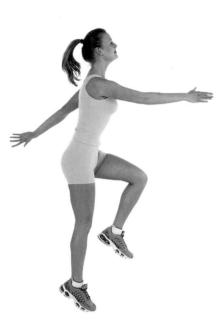

high-knees running

Pick your knees right up as you jog so that your thighs are parallel to the ground and you are jogging almost vertically.

lunge jumps

1 Assume the initial lunge position (see step lunges, above left), then push upwards from this position into a jump. Land back down into the lunge, going through the feet and bending your knees so that there is no jarring on the legs. Change legs and repeat.

2 A variation is to change your legs while in the air as you leap upwards from your lunge jump, so that you land with your other foot in front.

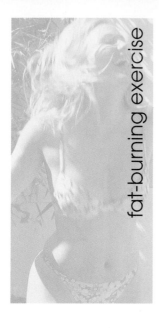

fat-burning exercise

aerobic exercise: pyramid circuit training

This circuit consists of six 'activity stations', giving you a range of different exercises that will keep your heart rate raised. Using the pyramid method as explained in the box opposite, perform each activity for 30 seconds before moving on to the next station and run a short distance between each level of the pyramid. This aerobic circuit should take 25–30 minutes if performed twice.

25–30 mins

good for: fat-burning; improving stamina; toning stomach and back muscles

++ extra fit: perform each activity for 45 or 60 seconds

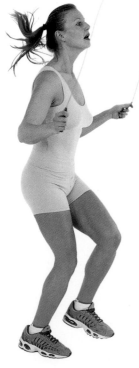

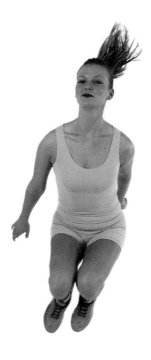

station 1: rope skipping

Skip at a comfortable pace, keeping your knees bent at all times and lifting your feet only very slightly using your hamstrings.

station 2: side-to-side jumping

Place a ball on the ground and jump over it from side to side.

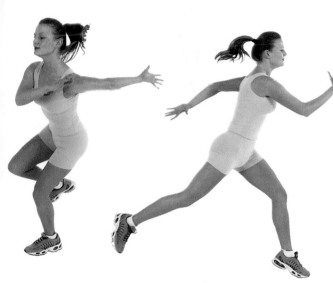

how does pyramid circuit training work?

A great way to work out, pyramid circuit training involves choosing six activities, each of which you perform for 30 seconds at a time, and an exercise break – in this case running 10 metres (10 yards) and back.

Start the session at the top of the pyramid with station 1 (skipping for 30 seconds), followed by the running exercise break. Then move down to the next level, where you perform the activities at stations 1 and 2 for 30 seconds each before repeating the running exercise, and so on down the pyramid. This type of circuit allows you to know precisely what you have done. By the end of the session you will surprise yourself at how many repetitions you have done in total.

station 3:
hopping

Hop on the spot, first with one leg then with the other.

station 4:
bounding

Start by jogging with large paces. As you jog, push hard off each foot so that you are spending longer in the air between each step.

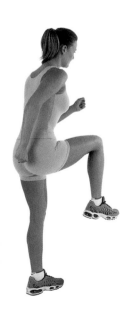

station 5:
stepping

Step on to a step bench then step back down at a comfortable pace.

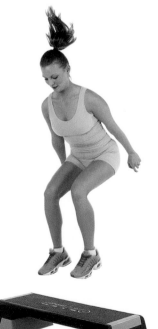

station 6:
jumping on to a step bench

Repeatedly jump with both feet together on to the step – rather than stepping up on to it – then step back down.

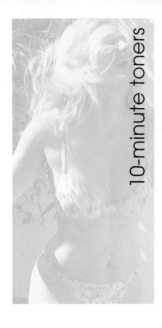

10-minute toners

10-minute bum toners

Many women are obsessed about the size of their bottoms. One of the problems with bottoms is that their muscles don't get much use in everyday life. Improving your posture will be a good start at waking those muscles up, while the following exercises will strengthen them, thereby lifting and firming the buttocks.

10 mins

good for: strengthening, lifting and firming the buttocks
++ extra fit: do more repetitions and perform the toning exercises every other day

back leg lifts

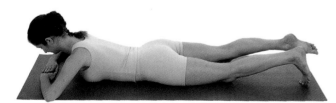

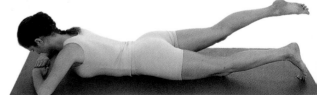

1 Lie on your front, resting on your elbows. Bend your left leg slightly and keep the foot flexed. Raise the right leg and stretch it to its full extent, pointing the foot. You should be able to feel the leg muscles working right into the buttocks.

2 Do 16 lifts each side then repeat another 16 times with the foot of the straight leg flexed.

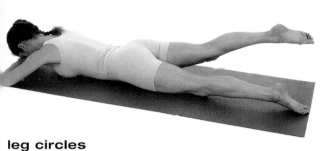

leg circles

Lie flat on your front, your face on your arms. Raise one leg straight behind you and make 16 little circles with your pointed foot, clockwise and then anticlockwise. Repeat with the other leg.

leg stretches

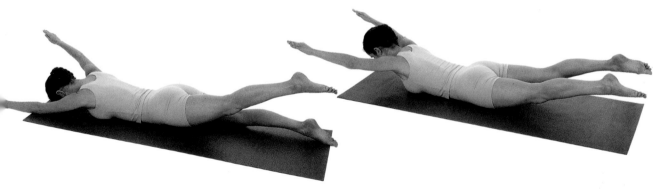

1 Lie face down on the floor, arms and legs stretched, feet about hip-width apart. Pull up your abdominals so that there is enough space to slide your hands between your stomach and the floor. Try to keep that pulled-up feeling throughout this exercise. Stretch out your left arm and right leg simultaneously, feeling the stretch right through your body – the stretch should lift your arm and leg about 15cm (6in) from the ground. Repeat with the opposite arm and leg. Do the exercise 8 times on each side.

2 Now repeat 8 times more with both arms and legs stretching at once.

buttock awareness

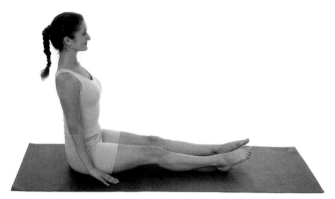

1 Sit on the floor, your legs stretched out in front, feet pointed. Your back should be perfectly straight, your arms beside you and hands on the ground. Pull your buttock muscles tight beneath you – you should find you are sitting about 5cm (2in) higher! Do this clenching and releasing 16 times.

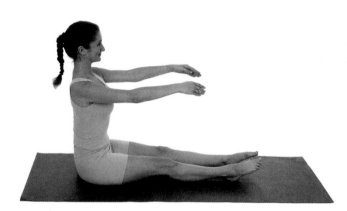

2 Now, with your buttocks clenched and your arms straight out in front of you, point your feet.

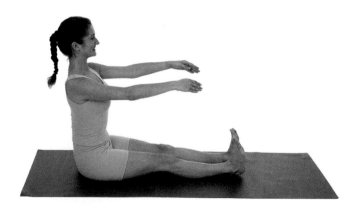

3 Now flex your feet. Point and flex your feet 16 times.

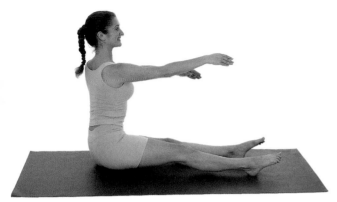

4 Finally, point your feet again and, sitting tall, move the left leg from the hip as if you are walking on your buttocks.

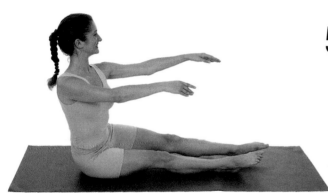

5 Alternate your legs so you walk 8 'steps' forwards.

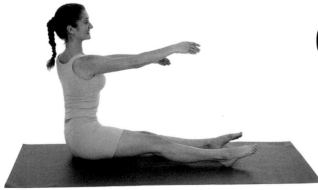

6 Now, alternate your legs so you walk 8 'steps' backwards.

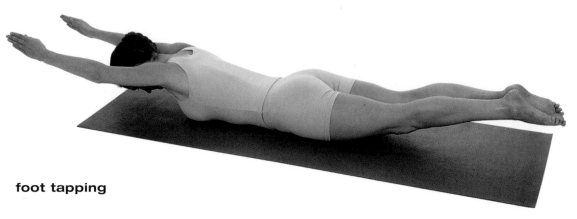

foot tapping

Lie face down on the floor and stretch out your arms and legs, with your head and chest off the floor as well. Tap your feet together, working up to 50 taps.

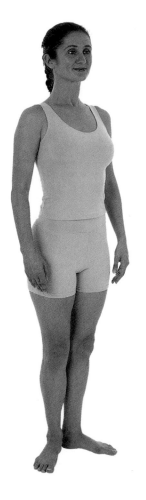

turn-out

Stand up very tall, your upper body relaxed and your back absolutely straight. Turn out your legs from the hip sockets very slowly so that your feet form a 'V' shape. Don't take your feet too far – your knees should be over your feet at all times, not rolling inwards. Then, at the same slow pace, draw your feet back to a parallel position. This exercise works the muscles of the buttocks and the inner and outer thighs. Repeat for 16 complete movements.

deep pliés

The more slowly you do this exercise, the more effective it is. You may need to hold a support such as a chair back to one side to help you balance.

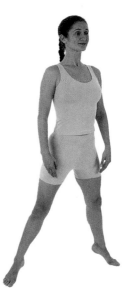

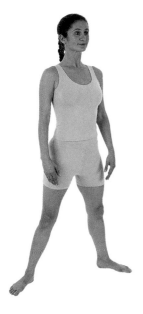

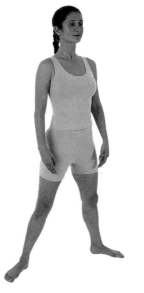

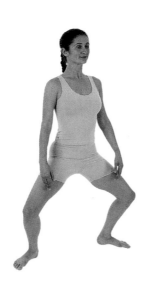

1 Stand tall with your feet about 45cm (18in) apart, your legs turned out from the hips without trying to over-extend the turn-out in the feet or ankles.

2 Keeping your back straight, drop your tailbone down towards the floor, bending your knees but without taking your heels off the floor.

3 Squeeze your thighs together to straighten, pulling up the muscles in your buttocks and the backs of your thighs.

4 Keep on squeezing so hard that you rise up on to your toes. Come down in one slow, smooth movement and bend the knees into another deep plié. Repeat the whole sequence 4 times in all, changing sides after 2 if you are keeping your balance by holding a chair back.

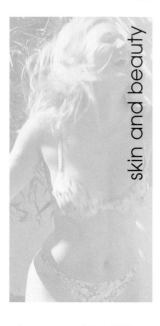

skin and beauty

shifting cellulite

Cellulite is the lumpy, chunky tissue, commonly seen in women of all sizes and ages. Even slim women can have cellulite, but it is undoubtedly more likely the older and more overweight you are. It is simply fat, which is packaged differently in women than in it is men thanks to the structure of female fat cells. It tends to appear where there is naturally more fat on the female figure – around the bottom, thighs and hips – and gives the skin the appearance of fleshy orange peel.

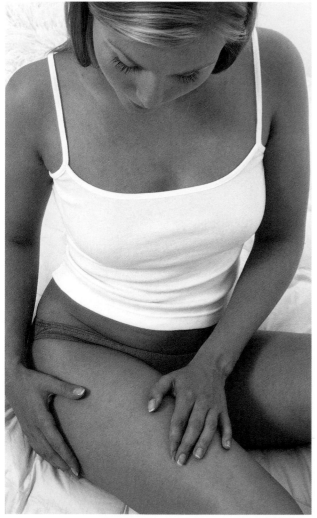

formation of cellulite

Cellulite forms gradually as a result of water retention, bad circulation and an unhealthy diet. The dimpled look is due to the fact that, unlike male fat cells, female fat cells are tall and pointed and extend upwards so are more likely to be seen protruding against the skin. The fat cells are held together by a network of fibres that are nourished and cleansed by body fluids. Poor circulation (or drastic dieting) can result in a slowing down of this cleansing process and an accumulation of waste materials that thicken and harden into immovable 'pockets' of fat. In time the skin loses its elasticity and the cellulite becomes more prominent.

combating cellulite

Anything that improves blood and lymph flow, and therefore elimination of toxins, can help in the battle against cellulite. Thus a healthy diet (which involves consuming less 'toxins'), a good intake of water and regular exercise are the main keys to fighting cellulite. In addition, exfoliation (see page 42), massage and skin brushing (see page 72) techniques all help improve circulation and the appearance of the skin.

salon treatments

Other remedies that claim fat-busting results include highly potent seaweed 'wraps' and all-over mud packs, both of which are salon treatments. Another salon treatment involves the use of a hand-held suction pump to massage the skin and stimulate lymphatic flow, thereby encouraging drainage and the removal of metabolic waste products. Also available are topically applied creams and lotions, as well as pills, which claim to help improve the skin's general texture and appearance by working on the sub-dermal layer of fat and improving the elasticity of the skin.

anti-cellulite massage

5 mins	**good for:** improving appearance of cellulite **frequency:** massage twice every day

Massaging areas of cellulite once or twice a day will improve blood and lymph circulation and minimize the appearance of the hard fatty lumps.

Stand in front of a mirror to make sure you treat all the areas of your body that suffer from cellulite. Apply a moisturizing cream or vegetable oil to the area to be massaged, so that your hands can glide smoothly over the skin. Massage firmly but not so hard that you hurt or bruise yourself. Use your thumb and four fingers to grip the skin and fatty layer beneath it then knead in small circular movements as though working with dough. Then massage across the skin using the base of the palm of your hand, working in long, sweeping strokes towards the heart.

Alternatively, try a special hand-held massager, which must be used with an oil or lotion to avoid friction and broken thread veins.

fight that cellulite

- **Improve your circulation with massage, skin brushing, exfoliation and exercise**
- **Drink more water to help reduce water retention and eliminate toxins**
- **Reduce your intake of salt, chemical food additives, caffeine and alcohol**
- **Take plenty of exercise: exercise helps to improve circulation and eliminate toxins; improved muscle tone will enhance the appearance of existing cellulite**
- **Take natural dietary supplements to help improve circulation and detoxify your system**

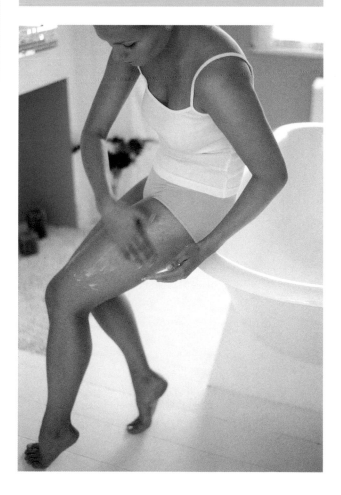

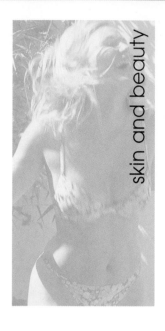

skin and beauty

skin brushing

Giving your body a firm brush all over on a daily basis boosts your circulation and helps to break down stored fatty deposits. As a result, skin brushing has a beneficial effect on areas of cellulite and can also help eliminate toxins from the body during the detox programme outlined in week one. In addition, the gentle massaging motion of the bristles makes the skin glow by removing the top dull, dead layer of skin and encouraging new cells to regenerate.

technique

Skin brushing is a simple technique for which you need only a loofah or a body brush (with natural rather than synthetic bristles) and a long handle or strap so that you can reach your back and buttocks. You need a much softer brush, or a flannel, for the face.

Skin brushing is carried out on dry skin. Start at your feet and work up your body, finishing with your face. Brush more gently where the skin is thinnest and always brush towards the heart. Brushing the whole body in this way will take between 3 and 5 minutes, depending on how many strokes you give to each area. It is best to brush before a bath or shower so that the dead cells are washed away.

Skin brushing is best done in the morning as the acceleration of blood flow is quite invigorating. The difference in your skin should be quite visible after just a few sessions – it will become very soft and develop a rosy glow.

5-minute skin brushing routine

Make sure the room is warm and there are plenty of towels. Undress, and sit comfortably so that you can easily reach your feet and lower legs.

5 mins

good for: boosting circulation and removing dull old skin cells
frequency: repeat every day

bikini-fit reasons for skin brushing

- Stimulates blood and lymph flow
- Helps eliminate toxins from the body
- Removes dead skin cells
- Encourages new cells to regenerate
- Stimulates production of sebum
- Helps combat cellulite
- Results in smooth glowing skin

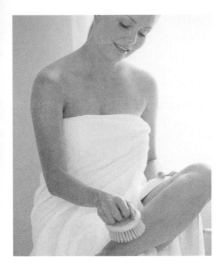

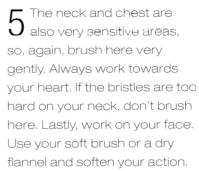

times, using long, rhythmic strokes. Brush your buttock area as far as your waist. Now repeat the whole procedure on your right leg, starting again with the sole of your foot. Starting from the top of your buttocks, and always moving in an upward direction, brush the whole of your back several times all the way up to your shoulders.

1 Take the brush and begin with the sole of your left foot. Use firm, rhythmic strokes to cover the sole several times. Next, brush the top of your foot, brushing up towards your ankle. Then go on to your lower leg, making sure you cover the whole surface – shin and calf. Always brush in an upward direction.

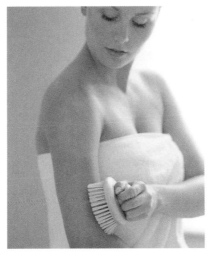

3 Next, brush your right arm. Start with the palm of your hand, move on to the back of your hand and then brush from your wrist up to your elbow, always in an upward direction and ensuring that the whole surface of your skin is brushed. Brush your upper arm, always working from your elbow towards your shoulder, again covering the whole surface of your upper arm.

abdomen, brushing in a circle, always in a clockwise direction. Cover the area several times but with less pressure than on your arms and legs. If it feels uncomfortable, stop.

5 The neck and chest are also very sensitive areas, so, again, brush here very gently. Always work towards your heart. If the bristles are too hard on your neck, don't brush here. Lastly, work on your face. Use your soft brush or a dry flannel and soften your action.

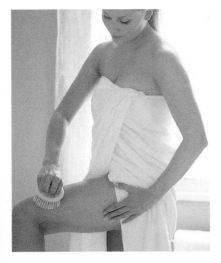

2 Stand up and brush the area from your knee to the top of your thigh. Make sure you cover the whole area several

4 Repeat on your left side, starting with your hand. Then, very gently, brush your

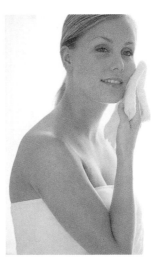

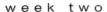

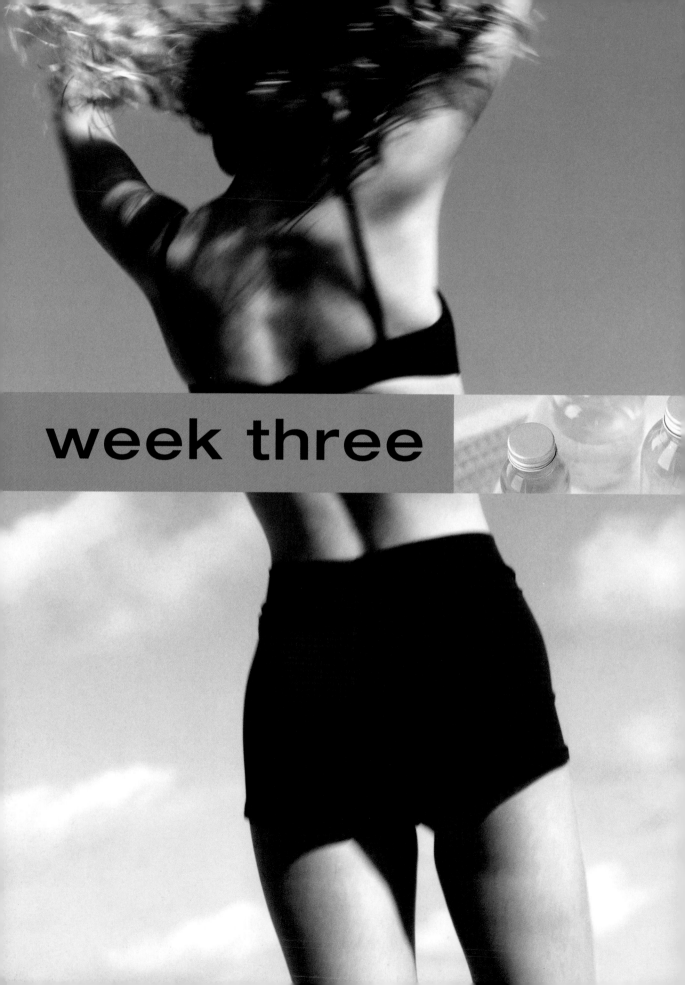

week three

Nutritious food and a healthy lifestyle are the key to beauty as well as good health and bags of energy. Supplement them with the techniques and treatments detailed in this chapter and throughout the book and you will certainly feel more beautiful and have the confidence to wear that bikini!

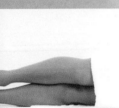

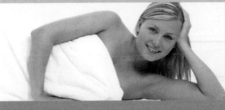

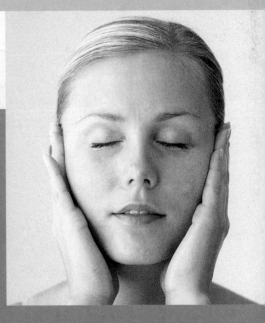

beauty

super skin and hair diet •
continued fitness workout •
thigh toners •
focus on your face •

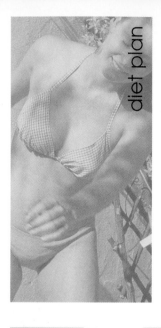

diet plan

wear what you eat

It is widely recognized that we are what we eat: our diet influences our health, how we feel and how we look. Just as our internal systems are affected by what we put inside our bodies so, too, is our only external organ, our skin. The skin needs a precise and complete supply of nutrients to regenerate, repair and defend itself. In effect, what you eat today you wear tomorrow. Even the most expensive skin- and haircare products cannot improve poor skin and hair without help from your diet.

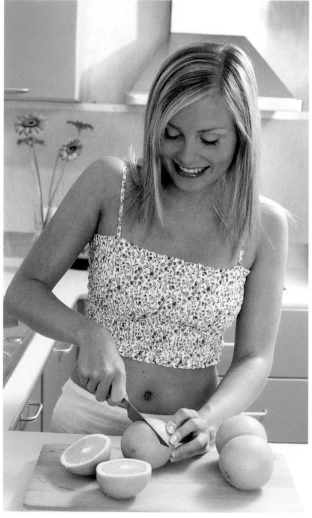

feeding your skin

If you have been making the changes to your eating habits advised in week two you will already be doing your skin good. Regularly consuming too many pre-packaged foods, which lack the nutrients that your skin needs, will result in a pasty complexion and lifeless hair. On the other hand, eating fresh fruit and vegetables, oily fish and low-fat dairy produce will do the opposite. You are more likely to have younger-looking, rosy smooth skin and shiny hair. As far as the skin is concerned, there are two groups of nutrients that are crucial to keeping your skin looking young – antioxidants and essential fatty acids (EFAs).

change your lifestyle

Beauty truly does come from within. Just as an unhealthy diet causes both your hair and skin to suffer, so too does an unhealthy lifestyle. Tiredness, stress, smoking and alcohol all deprive your body of nutrients and energy in various ways and consequently take their toll on your appearance.

antioxidants

Antioxidants protect us against minor infections and serious degenerative diseases such as cancer and heart disease, as well as conditions that come with premature ageing. They perform a fundamental role in destroying free radicals. Free radicals are the electrochemically unbalanced molecules, continually generated within our bodies by chemicals (pollution, cigarettes, certain foods), too much sun and stress. In skin, the main victim of free-radical damage is the collagen, which becomes tough and leathery.

The key antioxidants are vitamins A, C and E. The minerals selenium, manganese and zinc, some of the B complex vitamins and certain enzymes and amino acids also have antioxidant properties. A group of flavonoids called anthocyanidins are another group of very powerful antioxidants.

essential fatty acids

There are two classes of EFA, known as omega-3 and omega-6, and it is the former that most affects skin condition. The body cannot make EFAs so they have to come from our food. They are found in oily fish and fish oils, nuts and seeds and their oils, wild organic meats, algae, home-produced eggs, prawns and soya beans. Ideally, EFAs should account for at least 15 per cent of our calorie intake.

A quick way of increasing your dietary intake of EFAs is to use sesame, rapeseed, walnut, soya bean or flax oils in the kitchen, or eat canned oily fish such as sardines, mackerel and salmon. At the same time, decrease your intake of saturated and processed fats as these compete with and cancel out EFAs in the body.

Upping your EFA intake will not make your skin greasier, since EFA molecules disperse rather than stick together like those in saturated fats, so they do not clog the pores in the same way.

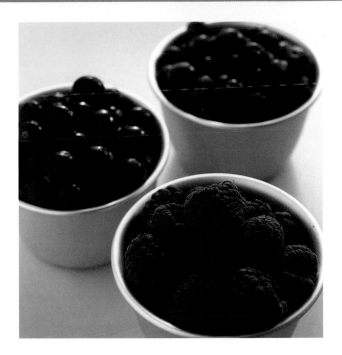

antioxidant-rich foods

Uncooked, highly coloured fresh fruit and vegetables are the best places to find antioxidants:

- Berries (strawberries, raspberries, blackberries, blackcurrants, redcurrants)
- Black grapes
- Brazil nuts
- Broccoli
- Carrots
- Cherries,
- Chestnuts
- Hazelnuts
- Kale
- Raisins
- Papaya
- Peas
- Peppers
- Prunes
- Spinach
- Sweet potatoes
- Tomatoes

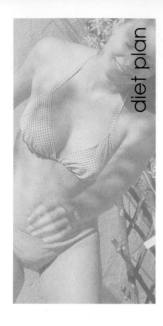

diet plan

super skin and hair diet

The skin, which includes the scalp and therefore the hair, is last in the queue of body parts to receive nourishment from our diet. Thus a poor diet means impoverished hair as well as skin. There are hundreds of vitamin-packed nutritional skin creams on the market, as well as vitamin and mineral supplements for skin, hair and nails. However it is far more effective – and certainly cheaper – to eat what the skin needs. In addition to the essential fatty acids (EFAs) described on page 77, the following nutrients are the best ones for healthy skin and hair.

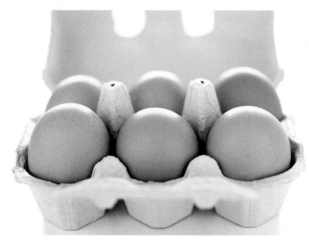

vitamin A

Involved in the formation of new skin cells, Vitamin A helps to keep skin supple and is also essential for healthy eyes and hair. Dry, flaky skin or scalp can indicate a deficiency of vitamin A.

best sources: Natural fats such as whole milk and butter, liver, oily fish, eggs. It can also be made in the body from beta-carotene (see below).

beta-carotene

This is the plant form of vitamin A, which the body converts into vitamin A as and when required. It protects against the ageing effects of ultraviolet light and boosts immunity.

best sources: Dark green vegetables (spinach, broccoli, kale, watercress) and orange-coloured fruit and vegetables such as apricots, mangoes, sweet potatoes, pumpkin, tomatoes.

vitamin B complex

This includes vitamins B1 (thiamine), B2 (riboflavin), B3 (niacin), B5 (pantothenic acid), B6 (pyridoxine), B12 (cobalamine), biotin and folate. The B vitamins help to release energy from the food we eat for skin metabolism, and have a role in maintaining normal skin function – keeping it moist and smooth. Signs of deficiency include:

• dermatitis (niacin, cobalamine, biotin)
• bloodshot eyes, cracks by the nose, lips or corners of the mouth and flaking skin (riboflavin)
• thinning hair and loss of hair colour (biotin)

best sources: Milk, oily fish, poultry, red meat, offal, eggs, bananas, soya beans, wholegrains, peanut butter, wheatgerm, breakfast cereals fortified with B vitamins.

vitamin C

The most potent of the antioxidants, vitamin C is essential for the production of collagen. Collagen is the elastic tissue in skin that declines with age. Smoking, stress and exposure to the sun can all drain vitamin C from the skin, leaving it vulnerable to damage. Dry, thin skin, easy bruising, splitting hair and bleeding gums indicate vitamin C deficiency. The vitamin C content of fresh produce diminishes with storage.

best sources: Citrus fruits, kiwi fruit, strawberries, blackcurrants, tomatoes, peppers, potatoes, peas, broccoli.

vitamin E

Probably the best-known skin nutrient, vitamin E is an antioxidant that works in tandem with selenium (see below), and which has the most powerful action against free radical damage caused by the sun. It also helps the skin to retain moisture, to maximize its use of oxygen and to produce new cells where the skin has been damaged. Premature wrinkles, pale skin, acne, easy bruising and slow wound healing may indicate a deficiency. Vitamin E tends to be lacking in our diet so a supplement may be necessary.

best sources: Vegetable oils, nuts and seeds, peanut butter, wheatgerm, wholegrains, avocados, sweet potatoes.

selenium

Selenium protects cells from free radical damage, and also helps to counter dry skin. It works with vitamin E to support the immune system, so can help fight infection before it breaks out on the skin's surface.

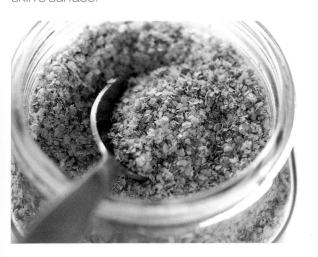

healthy hair

The nutrients that benefit hair are the same ones required by our skin – vitamin B complex, antioxidant vitamins, selenium, zinc and EFAs. In addition, drink plenty of water for silky, shiny hair; eat lean protein and green vegetables for the iron that encourages hair growth, and oily fish to encourage the flow of sebum, which gives hair its flexibility.

best sources: Cereals, meat, offal, seafood, cheese, eggs, mushrooms, brazil nuts, molasses, beans, wholegrains, wheatgerm.

zinc

Like vitamin C, zinc is vital to the manufacture of collagen. It also speeds up healing where skin has been blemished or otherwise damaged, and evens out pigmentation. It is vital to the immune system, helping to destroy infection before it surfaces on the skin. Lack of zinc slows down skin healing and can lead to stretch marks and stubborn blemishes. A dull complexion, white spots on fingernails, dry flaky skin and dandruff also demonstrate a zinc deficiency.

best sources: Seafood, red meat, offal, turkey, cheese, brewer's yeast, eggs, nuts, wholegrains, seeds, mushrooms, wheatgerm.

iron

Iron is particularly important for the formation of haemoglobin, the red pigment in blood. A pale complexion and prominent dark circles under the eyes may indicate a deficiency of iron in the diet, as can brittle nails that break easily.

best sources: Red meat, liver, seafood, eggs. Less absorbable is the iron found in leafy green vegetables, dried apricots, fortified cereals.

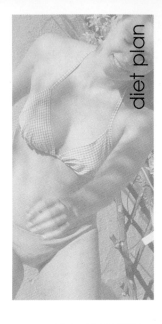

diet plan

rehydrate your body

During the course of a normal day, without breaking sweat, the average body loses at least 1.5 litres (2½ pints) of water through the skin, lungs, gut and kidneys. It has to do this to eliminate toxins – among them those that cause dark bags under the eyes and those that congregate under the skin to erupt as spots. Hot weather or physical activity will cause even more water to be expelled. At the same time as it is expelling water, the body also needs to produce water to burn glucose for energy (see page 102).

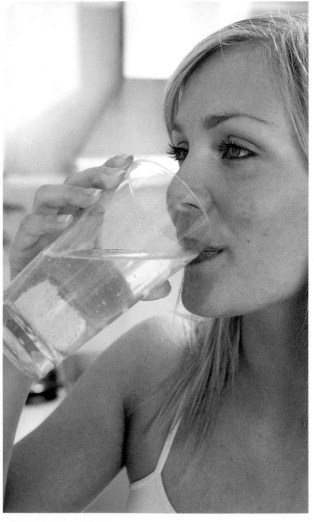

how much do we need?

The amount of water used and lost depends on our size and level of activity but, on average, we need to drink about 1.8 litres (3 pints) – or about 8 glasses – of *water* daily to function optimally. Few people drink anything like that quantity. Most of us are chronically dehydrated, without knowing it, and as a result suffer fatigue, headaches, indigestion and joint pain, the most common symptoms of dehydration.

Drinks like tea, coffee, beer and fizzy drinks do not count towards your daily intake as they still require filtration by the kidneys, whereas pure water does not. However you can 'eat' water, since most fruit and vegetables consist of about 90 per cent water. Grapes, melon, citrus fruit, peppers, cucumber and celery are examples of watery produce.

bottled or tap water?

In principle, there is good reason to swap tap water for bottled. Hundreds of chemical contaminants have been identified in tap water, the most common being nitrates, lead, aluminium and pesticides. But bottled water is not always the pure and simple substance it sounds.

Bottled water can be classified as table water, spring water or natural mineral water. Only the last is guaranteed to be from an unpolluted underground source. It is untreated and contains naturally occurring minerals, which have passed into the water as it flows through various layers of earth and rock to wells or springs, and which should be listed on the label. 'Spring water' is usually subterranean, too, but it does not have to be bottled on the spot and might have been treated to remove bacteria. 'Table water' is the least well defined and could be a mixture of water from many sources, including tap water. However, it has usually been purified and often has minerals added.

Bear in mind that spring or tap water is often artificially carbonated, a process that can cause carbon molecules to bind to minerals in the body and rob it of nutrients. Even the mineral content of true mineral water is small and not always a healthy balance. A water that is high in sodium, for example, will also have a mild dehydrating effect. Filtering your tap water is an alternative to bottled water and results in clearer-looking and fresher-tasting water.

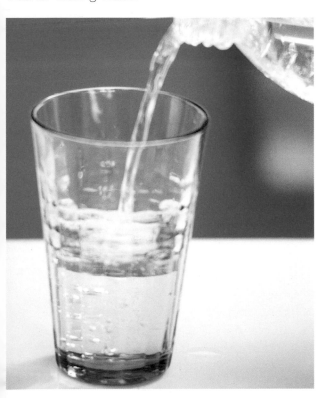

why you should drink more water

Keep your body in top condition by drinking at least 8–10 glasses of water per day. This will result in:

- Healthier circulatory system (more effective transport of oxygen and nutrients around the body)
- More effective flushing out of the kidneys (and therefore toxins), leaving fewer toxins to travel to the skin's surface
- Improved skin and hair condition (water keeps the skin cells plump and keeps lips hydrated). In people with dry-to-normal skin, it stimulates the sebaceous glands into producing more oil, which traps in more moisture. However, it does not make oily skin more oily
- Healthier digestive system (you are less likely to be hungry or constipated)
- Increased metabolic rate and raised energy levels
- Increased concentration and stamina
- Less susceptibility to stress, anxiety and exhaustion
- Slowing down of the signs of ageing, thanks to stimulation of the production of growth hormone from the brain's pituitary gland
- Reduced water retention and puffiness
- More effective fat-burning
- More powerful and flexible muscles in the face and elsewhere. Muscles should be three-quarters water and if they lose just three per cent of that they lose ten per cent in strength

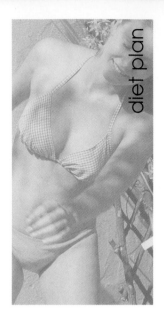

diet plan

looking lovely

We can make certain changes to our lifestyles to enhance our 'beauty assets' – that is, the appearance and health of our skin and hair. Drinking plenty of water (see page 80), which is paramount for both all-round health and our looks, is one of them. Other changes involve quitting smoking, limiting your exposure to the sun and reducing your consumption of alcohol, saturated fats and processed foods (typically loaded with chemical additives, extra salt, fat and sugar).

smoking and alcohol

Smoking thins the skin by around 40 per cent, so that water escapes much more easily. Similarly, alcohol dries out the facial skin and the scalp and, as a diuretic, causes the body to lose water quickly. It also makes red blood cells stick together and gums up the capillaries so that they can rupture, resulting in the formation of thread veins on the face. In addition, alcohol interferes with liver function, so facilitates the build-up of

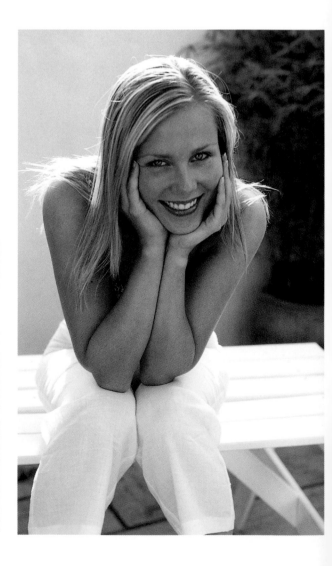

supplementary wisdom

Food is the best source of nutrients for your body's requirements, so if you eat healthily, vitamin and mineral supplements are not necessary, potentially even harmful.

People who may benefit from supplements, however, include women who are pregnant or breastfeeding or who suffer heavy periods, those who smoke or drink heavily, or who follow a strict vegan diet.

toxins, which are often pushed through the skin. Both alcohol and the chemicals in cigarettes rob the body of oxygen, vitamin C and other nutrients. The end result is that both alcohol and smoking can add years to the age of your skin.

dieting

Trying to lose weight has almost become a national pastime. Many people go about dieting the wrong way and so inevitably fail, often harming their skin in the process. The most common mistake is to cut right down on all fats. But as we have seen, the skin relies on a regular supply of essential fatty acids to keep it moist and pliable (see page 77). Yo-yo dieting (where you lose weight, regain it, lose it again and so on) has been shown to dry out and age the skin in the long term.

As outlined in week two (see pages 48–57), to lose weight but maintain a healthy body – and skin – diet at a sensible pace, include plenty of nuts, seeds and oily fish in your diet, and resolve to stick near your target weight once you have reached it.

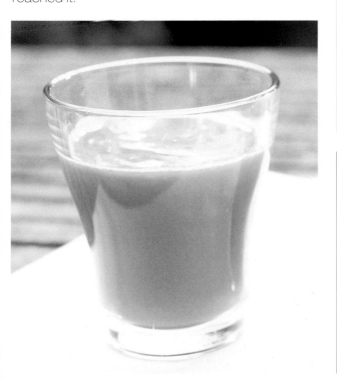

dos and don'ts for healthy skin

do...

- Drink plenty of water
- Eat seafood at least twice a week for the nourishing fish oils
- Use healthier fats like olive oil in preference to saturated fats
- Eat plenty of fruit and vegetables for a healthy dose of antioxidants
- Always wear a hat and sunscreen when in the sun

don't...

- Eat too much fried, smoked or barbecued food – these cooking methods destroy antioxidants
- Drink too much alcohol, tea or coffee, all of which dry out skin tissue
- Eat too much salt for the same reason
- Smoke, which robs the body of oxygen, vitamin C and other nutrients and prematurely ages skin
- Consume too much sugar, which hinders the body's natural detoxing process and can cause skin breakouts

smoothie for your skin

Blend together 1 small mango, ½ papaya, 1 tsp runny honey, 1 tsp lime juice, 50ml (2fl oz) orange juice and crushed ice for a smoothie that is packed with a healthy dose of skin-enriching nutrients – beta-carotene, vitamin C and vitamin E.

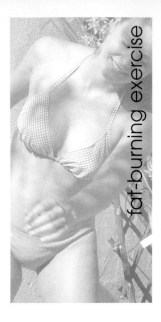

fat-burning exercise

muscle-building workout: combination weights

You will need to use light weights – two 1–2kg (2–4lb) weights – for this workout. Each of these moves is a combination of two exercises so you are doing twice the work in one move! Attempt each of these moves 10–15 times. Rest for 30 seconds between each move. Repeat the whole circuit 2 or 3 times.

exercise programme week 3

1 Warm-up (5–10 minutes) – see page 30
2 Muscle-building workout combination weights (10 minutes)
3 Aerobic exercise shadow boxing and/or speed play running (20 minutes) – see pages 86 and 88
4 10-minute toners (10 minutes) – see pages 36, 64, 90 or 114
5 Cool-down (5–10 minutes) – see page 34

10–15 mins

good for: shaping muscles (buttocks, back of arms, thighs); improving muscular endurance and strength
++ extra fit: do 15–20 repetitions of each move

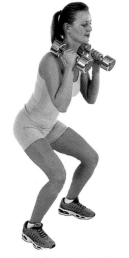

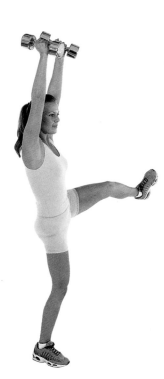

shoulder shack

1 Hold a dumbbell in each hand and rest your hands on your shoulders. Position your feet hip-width apart and pull in on the abdominals for support. Bend your knees slowly into the squat position, pushing your bottom behind you. Your weight should be over your heels and you should feel your buttocks taking the strain.

2 As you press back up to standing, lift one leg up as high as you can while pressing the dumbbells towards the ceiling. Return to the starting position and repeat with the other leg.

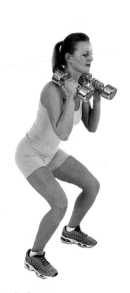
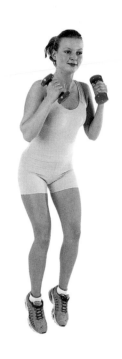

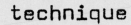

technique

Keep your breathing regular throughout these exercises and keep the abdominals tight to support the torso at all times. Focus equally on both the contraction (the beginning) and release phase of the movements.

slalom

1 Holding slightly lighter weights, use the squat position to jump and land.

2 Press your hips out to one side and then the other as if skiing down a fast snowy slope. Use your arms to push behind you as if holding ski poles.

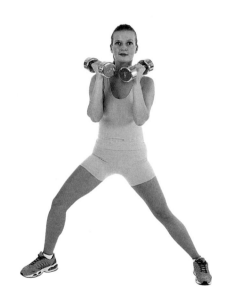

the perfect lunge

1 Stand with your arms raised to the sides, elbows at right angles, and a weight in each hand.

2 Step sidewards, bending your leg into a lunge position. As you bend the leg, press your elbows in to meet each other. Push back off the foot of the bent leg, opening the arms as you return.

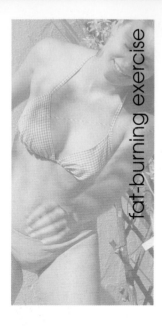

fat-burning exercise

aerobic exercise:
shadow boxing

Start by jogging from one foot to the other then add in some of the punches and moves below in 3-minute rounds. Have a 1-minute breather between rounds during which you should do 20 stomach curl-ups. Keep going for 20 minutes, bouncing on your feet at all times during rounds with no standing still.

20 mins

good for: fat-burning; improving stamina and coordination; muscle-toning
++ extra fit: increase each boxing round to 4 minutes

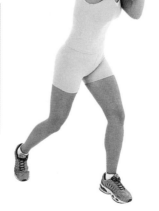

hook

The hook punch comes around the side. Bring your arm around in a semicircle with your arm parallel with the floor. This punch would land on the side of your opponent's head!

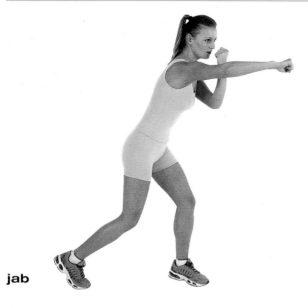

technique

Stand at all times in a pyramid position (take one step back with one leg and balance your weight) in relation to the object of your punches. This makes you a smaller target in real boxing. Keep your hands up as though to guard your face at all times.

jab

Start with both hands up near your face for protection. Extend one arm sharply and recoil it to perform the jab. You are aiming for your phantom partner's jaw!

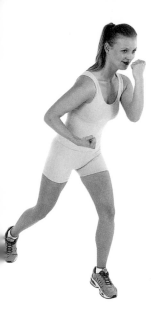

uppercut

The uppercut punch comes from low down, so bend your knees and swing the weight of your whole body upwards as you aim to punch up underneath your phantom partner's ribcage!

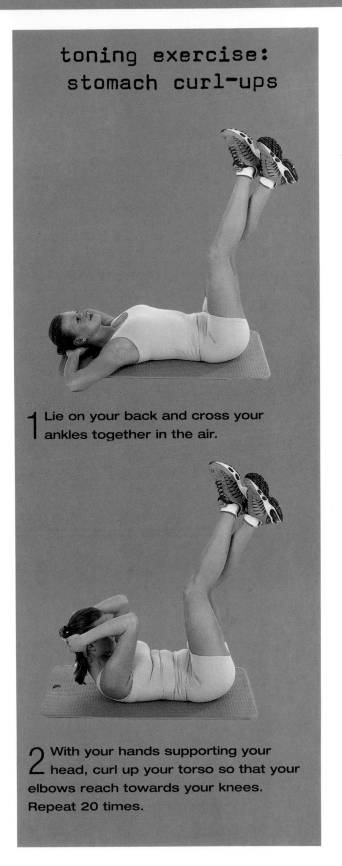

toning exercise: stomach curl-ups

1 Lie on your back and cross your ankles together in the air.

2 With your hands supporting your head, curl up your torso so that your elbows reach towards your knees. Repeat 20 times.

punch dodging

With your feet wide apart, use your whole torso and bend your legs to get low as the imaginary punches come at your head. Bob up and bob back down again as fast as you can.

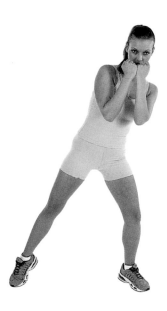

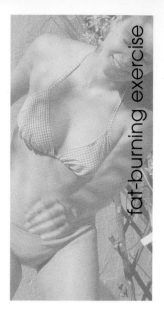

fat-burning exercise

aerobic exercise: speed play running

This running exercise is also known as *fartlek*, the Swedish word for speed play. It incorporates several types of running in a session – sprinting, running sideways, long-stride running, running 'vertically' by bringing your knees up to your chest, race/walking emphasizing lateral hip movement, walking on tiptoe to work the calves, or twisting from side to side while moving forwards. If possible, do this session on grass. Vary the programme below as you wish.

20 mins

good for: fat-burning; firming legs and hips
++ extra fit: make the steady runs between components shorter; increase the session length (see box far right)

technique

As with all running sessions, maintain a good posture. This means ensuring your foot lands in a heel–toe sequence. It also means trying to keep your weight over your hips and not sagging.

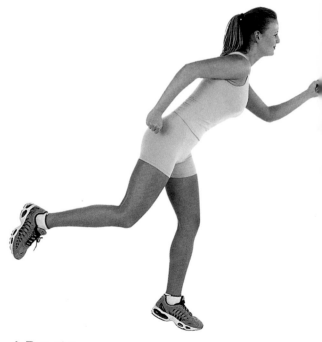

1 Run at a comfortable pace for 5 minutes then sprint until you reach the first person you see approaching you.

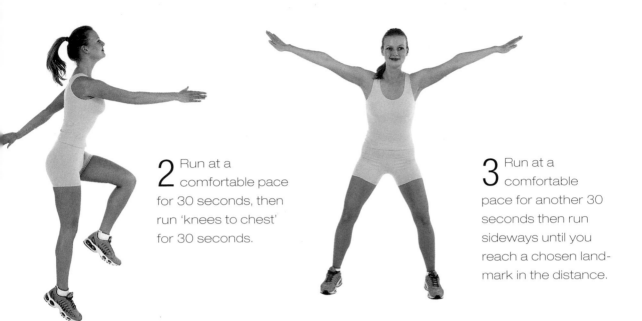

2 Run at a comfortable pace for 30 seconds, then run 'knees to chest' for 30 seconds.

3 Run at a comfortable pace for another 30 seconds then run sideways until you reach a chosen land-mark in the distance.

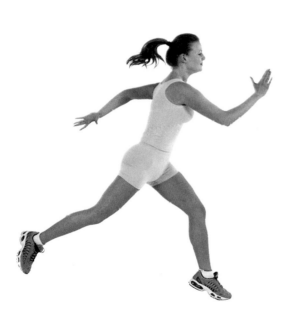

4 Run at a comfortable pace again, then race/walk until you reach a distant landmark. Continue the fartlek session along these lines. Play with your speed and your steps. Make sure the final 2 or 3 minutes are of a steady nature.

interval training

Interval training, which involves short bursts of higher intensity exercise as here, is one of the best ways to burn fat. If you want to work even harder during this workout, make the steady runs between components shorter (your recovery rate will improve as you get fitter), include more sprints, make the components last longer, or simply make the whole session last longer by doing more components. This is an excellent session for getting you out of your comfort zone.

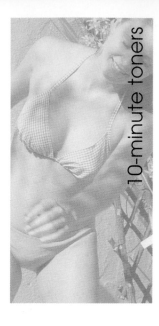

10-minute toners

10–minute thigh toners

Let's face it – nobody wants to be pear-shaped.
Bulging hips and thunder thighs are not exactly appealing.
Unfortunately, for most women, this is exactly where fat is
most likely to accumulate, often with the 'orange-peel'
effect of cellulite. Attack the problem, using diet and the
following exercises, which are designed to lengthen and
strengthen the legs. Where an exercise involves a leg
stretch, you should feel it pulled out to its full extent all
the way from the hip socket to the pointed toes.

10 mins

good for: strengthening and
toning the thighs; working the
stomach
++ extra fit: do more repetitions;
perform the toning exercises
every other day

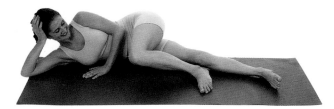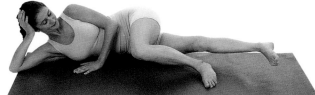

inner thigh lifts

1 Lie on your side, propped up on one elbow or
lying down flat along an outstretched arm.
Bring the top leg over the other one, bending your
knee, and place the foot on the floor. Extend the
lower leg and flex the foot.

2 Lift the lower leg about 15cm (6in) off the floor
16 times. Now repeat for another 16 with your
foot pointed. Repeat the whole exercise on the
other side with the other leg.

parallel pliés

These pliés strengthen the muscles at the front of the thighs, which not only gives your legs a firm, curved front but also protects the knees.

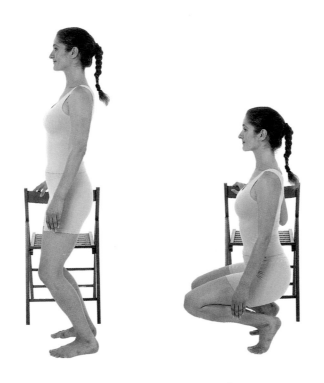

1&2 Stand tall with one hand resting on a chair back, feet together and facing forwards. Keeping your spine straight, bend your knees, dropping your tailbone smoothly down to the floor, only peeling your heels off the floor when you have to. Come back to standing and carry on upwards into a rise. Repeat for 4 pliés and rises on each side.

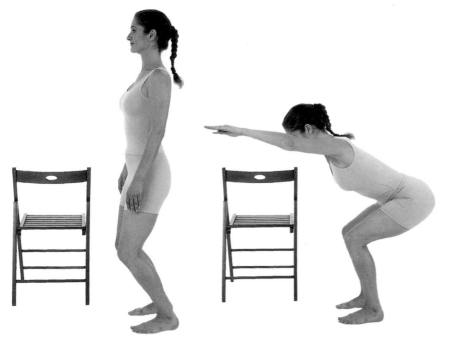

3&4 Move away from the chair but stand in the same lifted position. This time, as you bend, let your bottom stick out and aim to get your upper thighs parallel to the floor without lifting your heels. Swing your arms forwards as you go down to help you balance. Repeat 16 times.

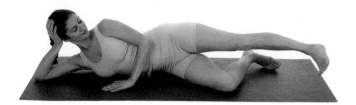

leg lifts

1 Lie on your side, either propped up on one elbow or lying down flat along an outstretched arm. Bend the lower leg and flex the foot so the heel is raised slightly off the ground. Flex the upper foot and push the heel away hard so the leg feels as if it is pulling out of the hip socket all the way through the exercise. Keep your back straight and your stomach held in.

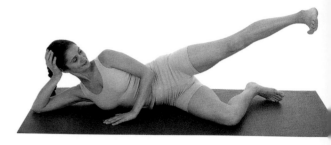

2 Raise the top leg and, from the raised position, do 16 small lifts.

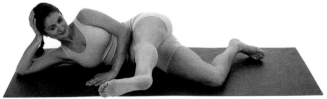

3 Lower the leg and take it forwards so that it is at a right angle to your body.

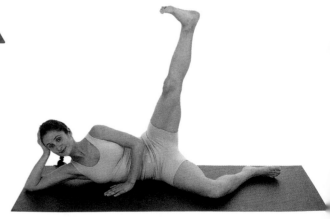

4 Keeping the foot flexed, raise it 16 times. Finally, in the same position, make 16 small circles clockwise then 16 anticlockwise. Repeat the whole exercise on the other side with the other leg.

double leg lifts

This exercise works the legs and the stomach very hard!

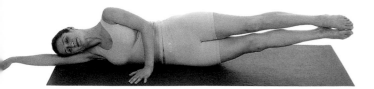

1 Lie on your side with your lower arm extended beyond your head. Point your feet to feel as if you are in one straight line from the tips of your fingers to the tips of your toes. Place your upper hand on the floor for balance. Slowly raise both legs at once, keeping them together. Lower and repeat 8 times.

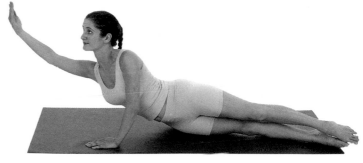

2 Now raise the upper body in a smooth, low curve, one arm outstretched. Lower and repeat 8 times.

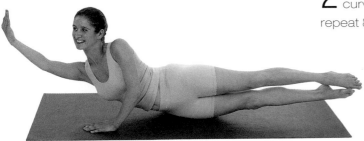

3 Finally, lift both your legs and your upper body at the same time and then lower them again 8 times.

leg sweeps

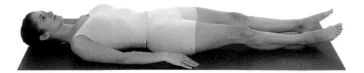

1 Lie flat on the floor on your back, with your knees and toes stretched and your stomach pressing down towards your spine.

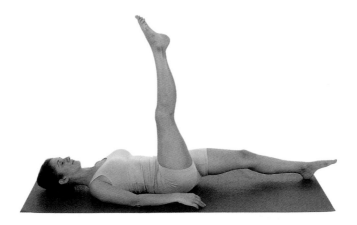

2 Slowly lift your right leg straight upwards and then down towards your chest as far as it will go, keeping it straight.

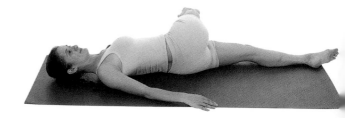

3 Now let it cross your body over the other leg and allow the weight of the leg to pull it down towards the floor.

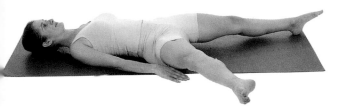

4 Return the leg across your body and down to the floor in a smooth circle. Alternating legs, repeat 4 times on each side.

leg kicks

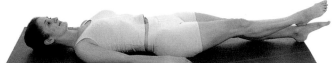

1 Lie flat on the floor on your back, with your knees and toes stretched and your stomach pressing down towards your spine. Lift your right leg, placing it so that it crosses over the left leg at the ankle.

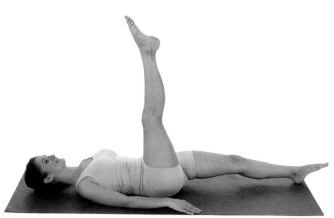

2 Lift it again very slightly and let it drop down on the left ankle to bounce straight upwards. Lower and place the left leg on top, bounce and kick. Repeat for 8 kicks on each leg, keeping the movement smooth and elongated and the small of your back on the floor.

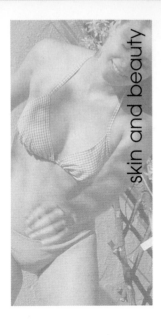

skin and beauty

face focus

When you first get up in the morning your face probably looks paler, puffier and more creased than usual, as a result of waste build-up thanks to the nocturnal slow-down in the systems that pump blood and lymph around the body. It is not only sleep that slows down circulation. During the day, lack of exercise, poor nutrition, shallow breathing and overexposure to pollution all slow the lymphatic and circulatory systems. Regular facial massage jumpstarts both blood and lymph flow, resulting in a healthy, pink glow.

what oil to use for massage?

Choose one of the following carrier oils, according to your skin type, to provide a fine, slippery surface for massage so that the skin is not pulled and stretched as you handle it:

• Dry or ageing skin: apricot, avocado, macadamia or wheatgerm oil
• Normal skin: almond, sunflower or sesame oil
• Oily skin: hazelnut, peach kernel or thistle oil

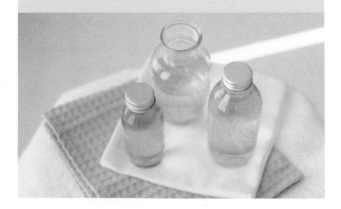

gentle massage

Pressing or squeezing any part of your body increases circulation to that area and the face, packed with small, sensitive muscles and nerve endings, responds particularly well to touch.

As well as improving the lymphatic system, which results in a resilient immune system and bright complexion, regular facial massage can be effective in countering wrinkles.

Both tension and age cause the tissue connected to the facial muscles to become less supple over time, resulting in wrinkles and frown lines. The gentle pressure of a facial massage can loosen up the facial muscles and allow them to learn to slide back into place more readily after being tensed. The cumulative effect is such that with repeated treatment your face will be left looking relaxed and younger.

The muscles of the face are extremely delicate so although a facial massage can be tremendously beneficial, do not massage too deeply or too frequently. In particular, sensitive skin, which is typically fair and dry, should be massaged with great care as it is more susceptible to the kind of surface damage that causes 'broken veins'.

4-minute facial massage

4 mins

good for: jumpstarting the circulation to brighten complexion
frequency: massage your face gently every day

You can do this after removing make-up using a carrier oil or while applying your moisturizing cream. Once you have memorized the routine it should take no more than 3–4 minutes, so try to do it every day.

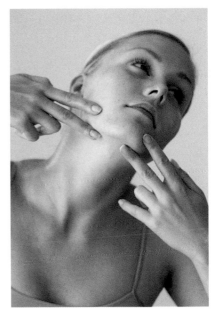

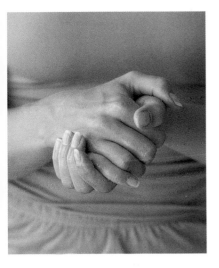

2 Using alternate hands, slide up your neck from the base to your jaw bone, turning the hands as necessary and working lightly over your windpipe. Cover your whole neck from ear to ear.

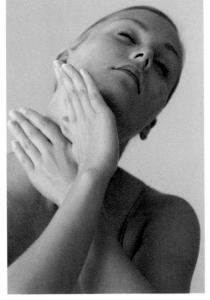

1 Pour just under 1 teaspoon of oil into one hand, rub it into both hands and apply the oil to your neck and face in long, upward and outward sweeping movements. Apply it very sparingly around your eyes, where the skin is most delicate, using the ring finger of both hands.

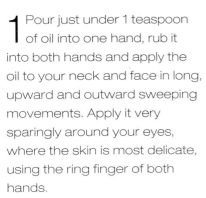

3 Using the first and middle fingers of each hand, slide firmly along your jaw line from your chin to the front of your ears. Your index finger should be on top of your jaw and the middle finger underneath.

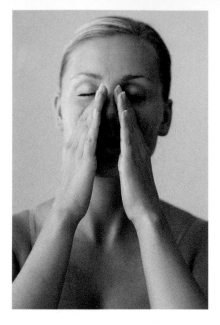

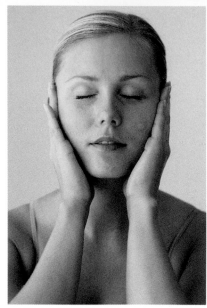

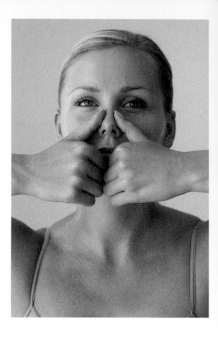

4 With your fingers together and hands pointing up to your brow, holding the fingers straight, press firmly with the edge of your hands either side of your nose. Hold for 3–4 seconds.

5 Release the pressure slightly and, rolling your hands on to your cheeks, slide your hands outwards with your index fingers stopping in front of your ears and apply a firm pressure. Hold for 3–4 seconds. Repeat.

6 With your fingers held in loose fists underneath your chin, slide both thumbs upwards symmetrically around the corners of your mouth, in under your nose, around your nostrils and lightly off over the tip of your nose.

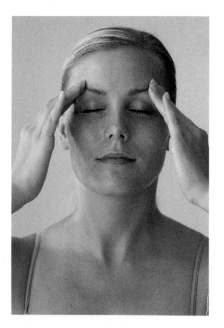

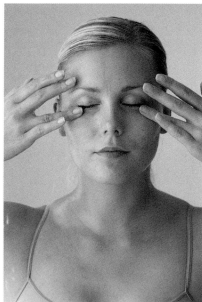

7&8 With the middle and ring fingers of each hand, starting at the inner corners of your eyebrows slide firmly outwards over your eyebrows and, using your ring finger only, trace very lightly inwards underneath your eyes.

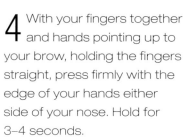

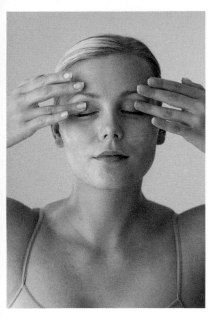 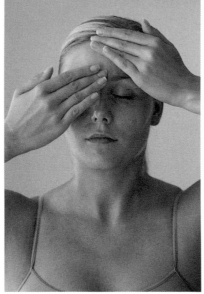 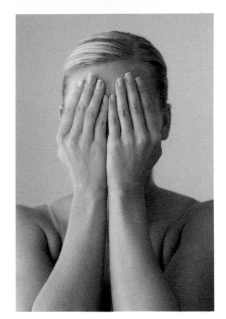

9 With the ring finger of each hand, slide lightly outwards over your closed eyelids and then lightly underneath each eye.

10 With your fingers together and the index fingers leading the way, alternately smooth the palms of the hands up to the hairline in a firm lifting movement, starting between the eyebrows and finishing at the hairline.

11 Close your eyes and, with the fingers together and using the whole of both hands slightly cupped to produce a gentle suction, apply a firm pressure to the face, holding for a second before releasing. Then, moving the hands outwards from the nose towards the ears, cover the whole face, moving the hands up and down to cover the area between the chin and hairline.

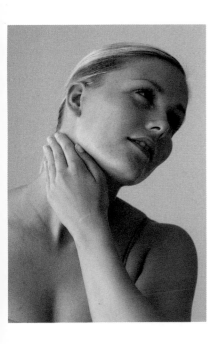

12 With your fingers together and using the whole of the hand, apply pressure with the right hand to the left side of the neck working from the base of the neck to the jaw but avoiding the windpipe. Repeat with the left hand, applying pressures to the right side of the neck.

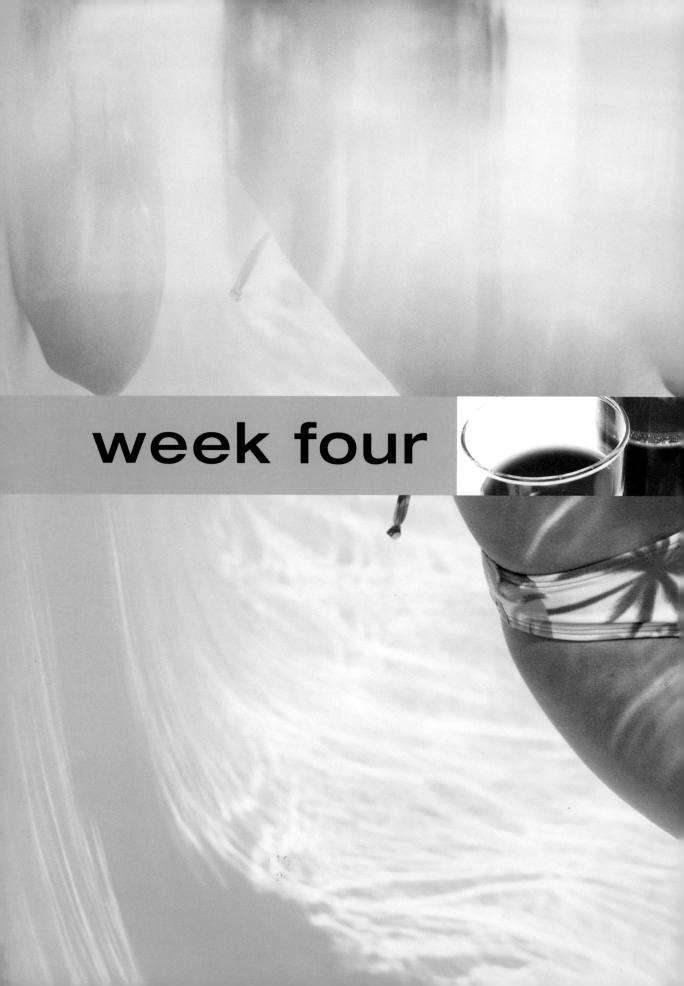

week four

If you have followed the bikini-fit plan, by now you will be feeling lighter, fitter and more healthy. Time for final preparations. By the end of this week, you will be ready to wow everyone – most of all yourself – with that slim, fit and healthy-looking bikini-clad body.

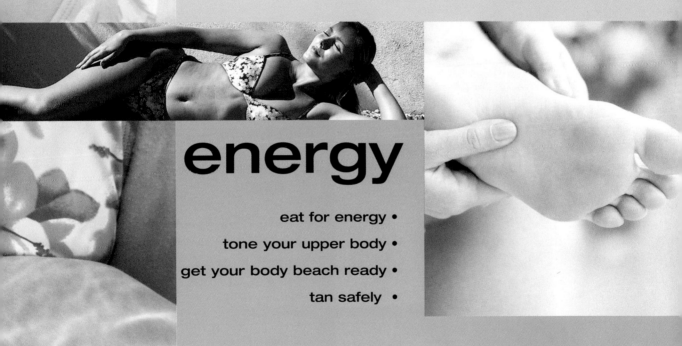

energy

eat for energy •

tone your upper body •

get your body beach ready •

tan safely •

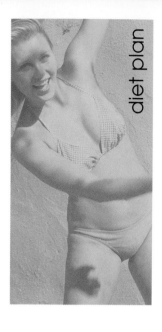

diet plan

be energy wise

We know from previous chapters that in order to function and stay healthy, our bodies need a regular input of energy in the form of calories provided by the food that we eat. But it is not just any old food that our bodies require. An unhealthy or irregular diet causes our internal systems to become sluggish and clogged with the toxins consumed, resulting in constant fatigue and lack of energy. To maximize vitality, therefore, our bodies need foods that boost the metabolism and keep blood sugar, and therefore energy levels, steady.

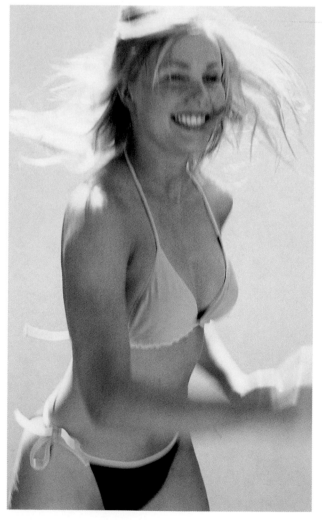

energy supply

Our food is made up of carbohydrate, protein and fat. Although some energy is supplied by fats and proteins, most of the energy in our diet comes from carbohydrate foods. This is because carbohydrates are more easily converted into the simple sugar – glucose – which is the body's preferred fuel for energy.

You cannot, however, simply increase carbohydrate intake to increase energy production, as this can upset blood sugar levels. Instead, eating at regular intervals and combining some protein and fat with carbohydrate at each meal helps keep blood sugar levels steady by slowing down the digestive process. It allows the body to 'burn' the carbohydrates as fuel and take the necessary nutrients from the other foods.

glucose – the body's fuel

All carbohydrates – both starches and sugars – release glucose into the bloodstream when digested. We should ideally have the equivalent of about 2 teaspoons of glucose dissolved in our blood at any one time. This blood glucose, or blood sugar, needs to be maintained at an even level for energy, concentration and alertness. The rate at which different carbohydrate foods release glucose into the bloodstream is measured on the glycaemic index (GI) and affects our energy levels.

The glycaemic index is a ranking of carbohydrate-rich foods from 0 to 100. The GI value ascribed to a specific food indicates the speed of its effect on blood glucose levels. The higher the GI, the faster the rise in blood glucose. Foods with a low GI release their sugars more slowly and should constitute the greater part of our diets. There is no easy way to determine the GI of a food. Generally speaking, low-GI foods are natural, less processed foods, and it is their high fibre content which helps to slow down the release of sugar into the bloodstream. Examples are wholegrains (such as brown rice, millet, oats, barley, quinoa), wholewheat pasta, dark rye bread, corn, beans and chickpeas, unsweetened yogurt and many raw fresh fruits and vegetables.

Fast-releasing, high-GI carbohydrate foods tend to be low-fibre, processed or sugary foods, which consist of easily digestible sugars that break down into glucose fairly quickly. Examples include sports drinks, jelly beans, chocolate biscuits, honey, sugary breakfast cereals, dried fruit, white bread and white rice.

the energy roller-coaster

Eating high-GI foods can flood the blood with too much sugar too quickly and result in an uncomfortable surge of energy. The body then releases a large dose of insulin to counteract the high blood sugar level. This response can bring your blood sugar level down too low, leaving you more tired than before and in need of another boost of energy. Such a roller-coaster of blood-sugar highs and lows, known as 'reactive hypoglycaemia', has a huge impact on both our energy levels and our moods. Continually raising and lowering blood sugar levels in this way can lead to severe health problems over time. The best way to moderate the effect of high-GI foods on blood sugar is to combine fast-releasing carbohydrates with a protein.

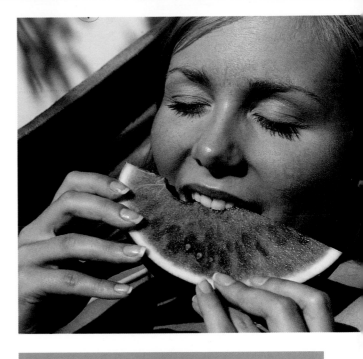

avoid sugar highs and lows

Eating a bar of chocolate or biscuits gives your body an influx of refined sugar, which might provide a fleeting burst of artificial energy but will quickly leave you feeling more tired than you were before, as your body tries to correct the blood sugar imbalance.

Snack on grapes, cherries or an apple instead to raise blood sugar levels slowly and give you stamina. For a quick energy boost, eat a ripe banana.

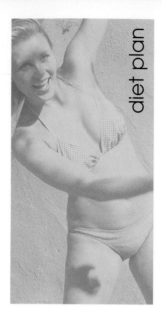

diet plan

eating for energy

Now that you know where your energy comes from, you can tailor your eating habits for maximum energy levels. Your body needs fuel every few hours to stimulate the metabolism and keep blood sugar, and therefore energy levels and moods, steady. So plan to eat three meals a day with regular snacks in between. At times when you need extra energy, avoid eating large, rich meals which require lots of energy for digesting and may slow you down. Instead, eat small simple low-fat meals or snacks throughout the day to keep your body sufficiently fueled.

breakfast

Because metabolism slows down during sleep your body needs a good input of energy in the morning to get it going again. Breakfast is therefore the most important meal of the day. If you really cannot eat first thing, be sure to eat something within the first 2 hours of waking. Avoid high-GI, refined carbohydrates like white sugar, white bread and sugary breakfast cereals. Instead, combine starchy carbohydrates (natural wholegrain breads and cereals) with low-fat protein foods to give your brain and muscles the energy they need for the first half of the day.

breakfast ideas: Egg (scrambled or poached) or beans on wholemeal toast; yogurt or silken tofu and fruit smoothie; wholegrain cereal with milk and fruit; porridge; wholemeal toast with peanut butter.

mid-morning or mid-afternoon snack

To maintain your energy levels throughout the day, avoid snacking on high-GI foods loaded with simple sugars. Instead, choose fruit, cereal or wholegrain bread with some low-fat protein to help you last until the next mealtime.

snack ideas: Boiled egg with wholemeal toast; rice cake/bagel/oatcake/wholemeal crackers/crispbread with toppings such as tuna, avocado, hummus, peanut butter or cheese; small packet of dried fruit and nuts; vegetable sticks with soured cream dip; orange slices and cottage cheese; low-fat yogurt; apple and a handful of nuts; low-fat smoothie.

top energy foods

- **Starchy carbohydrates** – wholegrains (brown rice, millet, buckwheat, oats, barley, quinoa), wholegrain/rye bread
- **Protein** – cottage cheese, eggs, nuts and seeds, oily fish, poultry, pulses, seaweeds, tofu, yogurt
- **Vegetables** – artichokes, asparagus, beetroot, broccoli, brussels sprouts, carrots, cauliflower, mushrooms, peppers, spinach, sweet potatoes, turnips, watercress, yams
- **Fruit** – apple, avocado, banana, berries, mango, papaya, pear, pineapple

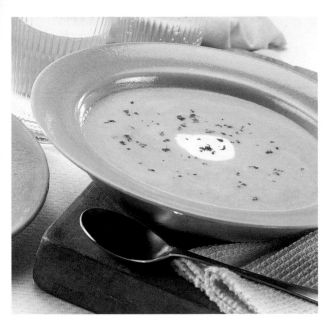

dinner

If you need to stay alert for the evening, as for lunchtime, choose low-fat proteins and vegetables and avoid too many carbohydrates. Otherwise, you can indulge yourself a little with other foods, but always remember the recommended food group servings (see page 50).

dinner ideas: Grilled fish, baked potato and green vegetables; chicken and mushroom risotto; grilled steak and salad; prawn and vegetable kebabs and rice.

bedtime snack

Don't eat high-sugar or fatty foods, which take time to digest, before turning in – choose carbohydrates instead to help you fall asleep.

snack ideas: Low-fat yogurt; skimmed milk and banana; wholemeal crackers; fruit salad.

lunch

Low-fat protein is a good choice for lunch as it increases the production of brain chemicals called catecholamines, which will enhance alertness and energy levels throughout the afternoon. Avoid eating saturated fatty foods and big heavy meals at lunchtime – both require a lot of digesting, which saps energy. Similarly, a large helping of carbohydrates may not be a good idea at lunchtime as carbohydrates increase the level of serotonin in the brain and make you sleepy.

lunch ideas: Hearty soup (vegetables, chicken, beans) and wholemeal roll; hard-boiled egg and tuna salad; turkey salad wholegrain sandwich; grilled fish and vegetables.

low-fat protein

Eating low-fat protein for breakfast or lunch avoids hunger pangs between meals as it fills you up for longer. Low-fat yogurt, tofu, lean meat, chicken, turkey, fish, low-fat cheese, cottage cheese and skimmed milk are all good options.

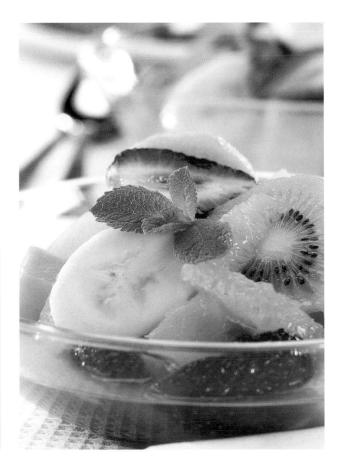

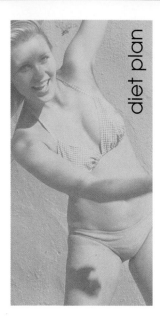

diet plan

be energized

By making a few changes to your lifestyle, in particular eating and drinking wisely, you can up your energy levels considerably. Other factors include getting enough sleep, managing stress, which seriously saps energy levels, and increasing your level of activity. Exercise may initially wear you out but it actually leaves you feeling more energetic and revitalized thanks to the rush of endorphins your body releases when you exercise.

eat for energy

As well as eating regularly (see page 104), avoiding processed and fatty foods – which strain the body's own detoxifying systems – will help keep energy levels high. Many tips on eating for energy are simply healthy eating habits and ways to lose weight, as outlined on page 50. For example, replace white sugar with honey and use cold-pressed olive oil instead of saturated oils.

when to eat

What time of day you eat can affect how your body uses the food you consume. Ideally, your evening meal should be the smallest of the day, or at least eaten early in the evening, so that the food is not left in your stomach to be digested overnight when your metabolism automatically slows down.

After eating a meal, allow 1–4 hours (depending on the meal size) before exercising to avoid experiencing sluggishness and cramp while your body is trying to do two jobs at once (digestion and exercise). Just before, during and after exercising, eat a small snack of a low-fat high-GI carbohydrate food, such as a low-fat sandwich, dried or fresh fruit, or a smoothie, which provides energy but is easily digested.

factors that deplete energy

- **Dehydration**
- **Unhealthy food choices**
- **Irregular eating**
- **Overeating**
- **Caffeine**
- **Nicotine**
- **Alcohol**
- **Stress**

drink for energy

Dehydration can affect your energy levels, so increasing your intake of water (see page 80) will banish feelings of fatigue and dramatically increase your vitality. Never consider a cup of tea or coffee as a quick 'pick-me-up'. The caffeine provides only short-term energy and places unnecessary stress on the body by dehydrating it and interfering with its absorption of vitamins. Natural herb teas or green teas are energy-boosting alternatives.

get enough iron

An iron deficiency in the diet can cause a lack of energy. The best sources of iron in the diet are red meat, liver and eggs because this iron is most easily absorbed. Blackstrap molasses (available from healthfood shops) is another good source. The iron in fortified breakfast cereals, vegetables or added to flour is less well absorbed, but its absorption is helped by taking a source of vitamin C, such as orange juice or salad vegetables, at the same time. Caffeine inhibits absorption of iron, so avoid drinking tea and coffee around meal times. If you suffer heavy periods, an iron supplement may be necessary.

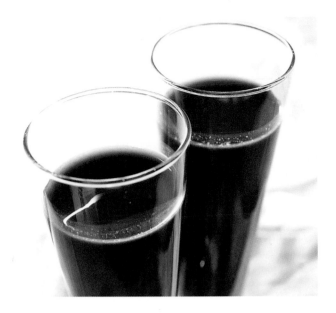

make yourself a smoothie

Smoothies are excellent energy boosters and are an energy- and nutrient-packed breakfast option. Experiment with quantities and various combinations of fruit, fruit juices, honey, spices, silken tofu, skimmed milk and low-fat natural or flavoured yogurts to suit your own tastes. Drink it as soon as you have made it.

For the simplest smoothie, blend a sliced banana with orange juice or with skimmed milk and/or low-fat natural yogurt to taste. Additional ingredients could include some fresh or frozen strawberries, canned peaches or dried apricots, or a sprinkling of grated ginger or nutmeg. A handful of porridge oats, soaked in milk, makes another good addition to smoothies.

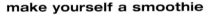

juice for energy

Juice together half a pineapple, a mango and a papaya for a wonderfully exotic and sweet energy booster, ideal for when you feel stressed or tired. Drink at once.

Another sweet-tasting, energy-giving option is to juice together 10 raspberries, 5 strawberries and 3 apricots. Whiz the mixture with 100g (4oz) low-fat natural yogurt and drink.

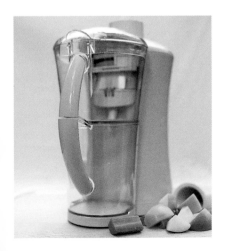
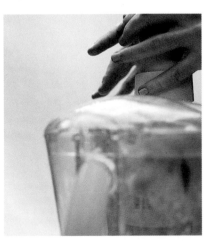
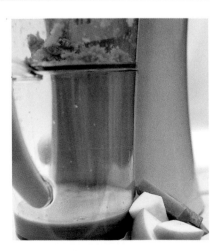

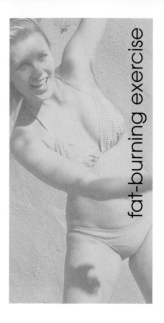

fat-burning exercise

muscle-building workout: mid-section weights

This workout involves pushing the muscles hard. You need to use dumbbells that are heavy enough to challenge you after 8 repetitions. If you use dumbbells that have add-on weights you can alter the resistance, either increasing or reducing weight as necessary so that 8 repetitions are the most you can manage.

exercise programme week 4

1 **Warm-up** (5–10 minutes) – see page 30
2 **Muscle-building workout** mid-section weights (10 minutes)
3 **Aerobic exercise** dance and/or stairs workout (20 minutes) – see pages 110 and 112
4 **10-minute toners** (10 minutes) – see pages 36, 64, 90 or 114
5 **Cool-down** (5–10 minutes) – see page 34

10 mins

good for: toning stomach muscles; improving muscular endurance and strength
++ extra fit: add extra weights as you become stronger over the weeks so that you can still handle only 8 repetitions

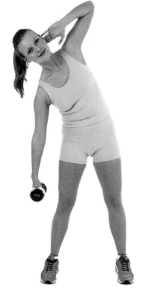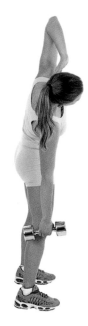

side bends

1 Stand with your feet hip-width apart and your knees slightly bent. Pull in on your abdominals and lift your chest. Grasp a weight in one hand and hold it at one side of your body. Now let the weight tilt you over to one side. Maintain this pose while you check your position. Check that you are not arching your back or bending forwards.

2 Now contract the sides of the abdominal area (the oblique muscles) to bring you back to the upright position. Do 8 repetitions of this 'tilt and return' on each side to tone the sides of the stomach.

cheating row

1 Step into a lunge position and lean forwards, resting one hand on your thigh. Let the other arm, holding the weight, hang down to the floor.

lateral raises

1 Stand with your feet hip-width apart and your knees slightly bent. Pull in on your abdominals and lift your chest. Holding a weight in each hand, and keeping your arms slightly bent and rounded, lift them out to the sides until they are parallel with the floor.

2 Hold this position momentarily then tip the end of the weights downwards and forwards slightly as if you are pouring from a jug. Slowly lower your arms with control, breathing freely throughout. Do 8 repetitions, focusing on the muscles that you are using at the sides of your torso.

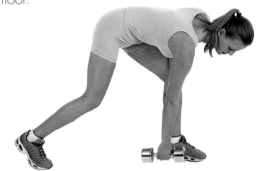

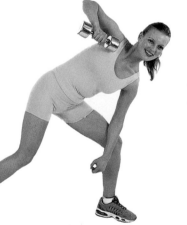

2 Pull up your arm, turning your body so that it faces to the side. Be sure to keep the supporting knee from twisting: the movement should be generated from the sides of the torso. Hold and release down. Repeat 8 times on each side.

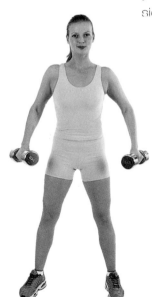

technique

With each of these exercises make sure that you are handling the heaviest weight you can for 8 repetitions only. If you can manage only 5 repetitions, the weight is too heavy. If you can manage 15 add a little more weight to your dumbbell.

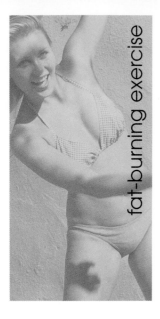

fat-burning exercise

aerobic exercise: dance workout

Keep dancing for 20 minutes! This is your freeform workout and your chance to be creative. You can make this workout as hard as you want. Put on a piece of music that you love and really get moving! You will probably find you are more stiff after this workout than any other. This is because you will have used muscles you didn't know (or had forgotten) you had!

20 mins

good for: fat-burning; working seldom-used muscles
++ extra fit: wear light wrist or ankle weights

challenge yourself

If you like a challenge, try this workout on another day wearing light wrist or ankle weights.

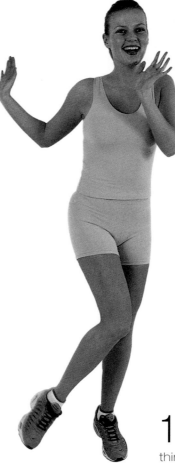

1 Start off by jigging on the spot. Now think of every dance move you've ever known and start adding them in! Move your hips, swing your arms and leap and turn about!

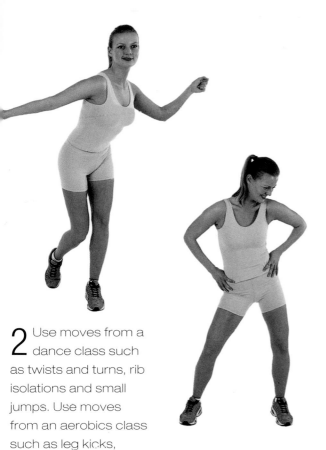

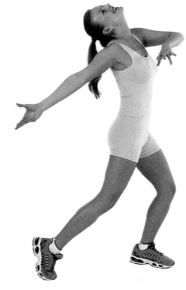

2 Use moves from a dance class such as twists and turns, rib isolations and small jumps. Use moves from an aerobics class such as leg kicks, grapevines and star jumps.

3 Use moves from the Lambada scene such as hip rotations, back leans and shoulder shimmies. Use moves from partner dances such as the waltz step, the Charleston and the cha-cha.

4 Use moves that you remember (or make up) from rock-and-roll movies and jive dances. Whatever you do, just keep moving and don't stop!

exercise time is time for you

- Don't miss a session because you think you haven't got time. For every hour you spend exercising, you will get back double in terms of the energy levels you will have for the rest of the day.
- Remember that time spent exercising will distance you from the stresses and excitements of your day and allow you time to think, relax and focus – or dream about your holiday!

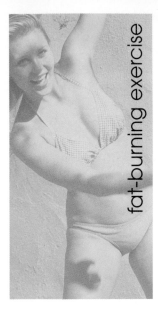

fat-burning exercise

aerobic exercise: stairs workout

You can get a good aerobic workout simply by using your stairs at home energetically. If you don't have suitable steps of your own, find some outdoor ones in a local park for this 20-minute cardiovascular workout.

20 mins

good for: fat-burning; strengthening heart and lungs
++ extra fit: carry or wear light weights while you work out

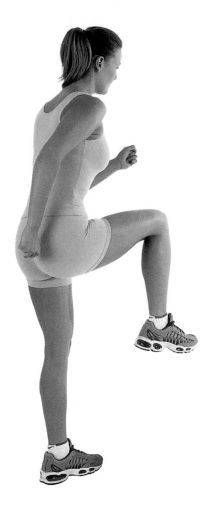

1 Run up and down the stairs 3 times to get warm.

2 Run up 1 step and back down. Run up 2 steps and back down, then up and down 3 steps and so on, until you have been all the way up and down the stairs.

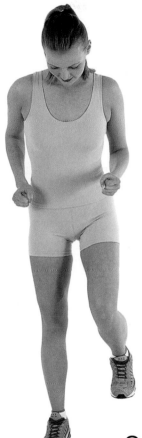

technique

Watch that your knees are in line with your toes as you step upwards. On the way down, pull up on the abdominals to support your back and step through the toes to the heel to protect your knees.

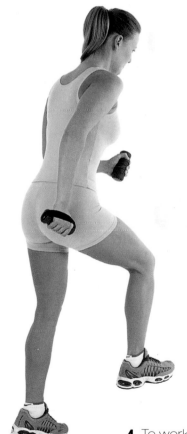

3 Then go up the stairs 2 – or even 3 – at a time, coming back down the usual way. When you get to the top of the stairs perform 5 small feet-together jumps. Finish with 3 trips up and down the stairs.

4 To work even harder, wear wrist weights or carry some light weights while you do this workout.

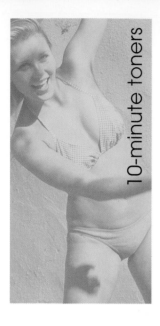

10-minute toners

10-minute upper body toners

More often than not, we concentrate on exercises for thighs, tums and bums and sometimes forget about our muscles above the waist. The following exercises are designed to remove tension in the neck and shoulders, improve posture and address particular problems such as flabby arms. Never let your shoulders hunch in tension or your spine slump. Keep a mental picture of a lifted, elongated spine, a long neck and a gracefully held head. There will be an instant improvement in how you look.

10 mins

good for: easing neck and shoulder tension; improving posture; toning flabby arms; firming your bosom
++ extra fit: perform the exercises every day

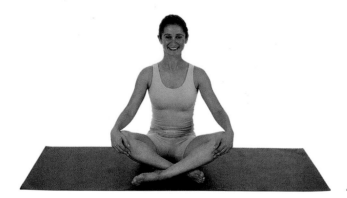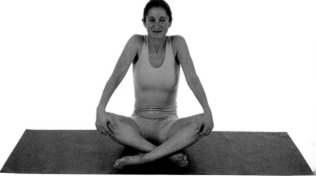

shoulder lifts

1 Sitting or standing with a straight spine and a long neck, feel your shoulders dropped right down into your back.

2 Now lift them as high as you can – right up to your ears – then let them drop down. Repeat 8 times.

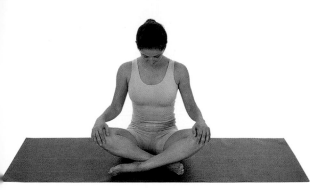

head rolls

1 Standing or sitting with a straight spine and
dropped, relaxed shoulders, let your head fall
forwards on to your chest.

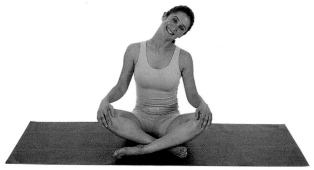

2 Very slowly, roll it around to the left until it is
parallel with your shoulder – make sure you
don't draw your shoulder up to meet it.

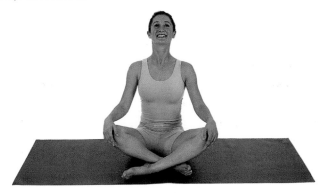

3 Continue round to the centre back then return
to your starting position. Repeat on the right.
Repeat the whole exercise 6 times.

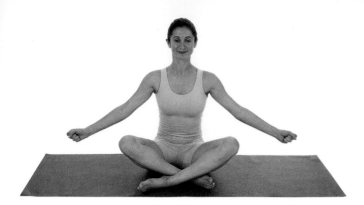

clenching fists

1 Sit cross-legged (or however you are most comfortable) with a straight back. Feel your body lifting up out of your waist and stretch your arms out low at your sides with your hands clenched into fists.

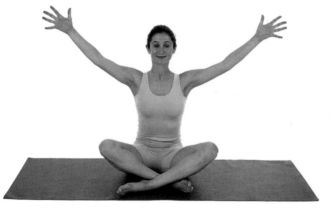

2&3 Fling your fingers out, stretching them as far as they will go. Repeat the clenching and stretching as you raise your arms, taking 8 flings to get your arms pointing straight up and another 8 to get back down again. Build up to doing the whole exercise 4 times.

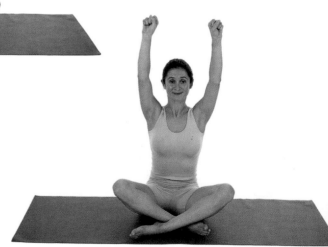

bosom firmer

The breasts themselves have no muscles but this exercise works on the pectoral muscles that lie beneath the breast tissue.

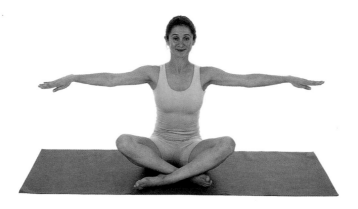

1 Sit cross-legged with your arms stretched out to the sides at shoulder level.

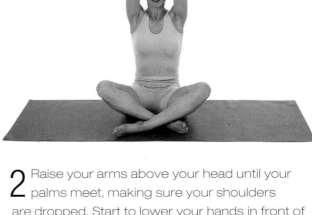

2 Raise your arms above your head until your palms meet, making sure your shoulders are dropped. Start to lower your hands in front of you, pressing them hard together as you do so. You should feel the pectorals working straight away, feeling almost as if they are pulling the arms down.

3 Lower your arms until your hands are in front of your breast bone, then take them out to the sides and repeat the whole sequence 4–8 times.

arm crosses

This works on both the upper arms and the pectoral muscles.

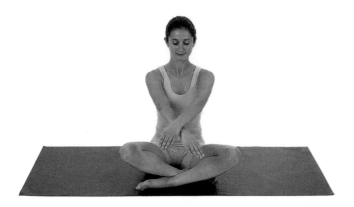

1 Sit cross-legged with your arms stretched out in front of you, crossed at the wrist and pointing towards the floor.

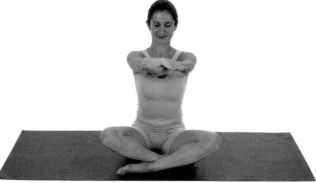

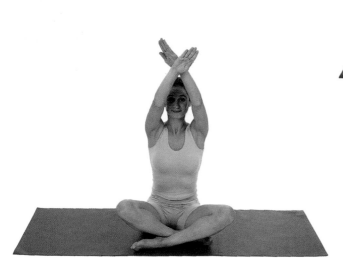

2 & 3 From here, start to raise the arms, crossing and recrossing them, alternating which arm is on top. Take 8 crosses to reach the top and another 8 to come back down. Make sure you look straight ahead and keep your neck long. Repeat 4 times.

flipper hands

This exercise is a really effective assault on flabby upper arms!

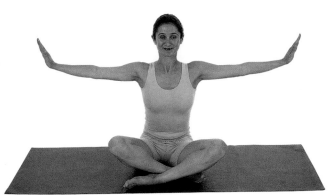

1 Sit cross-legged with your arms straight out to the side at shoulder level. Push away from the shoulders so that the arms are fully extended and flex the hands back, keeping the fingers straight so that you feel a stretch right along the underside of the arm.

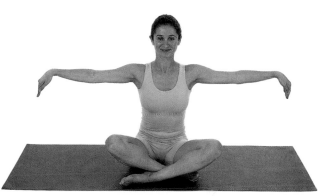

2 Now drop the hands and curl them under as far as they will go. This time, you should feel a real pull along the backs of the hands, wrists and forearms. Repeat the sequence 16 times, keeping the shoulders dropped throughout.

spot reduction is a myth

Unfortunately, you cannot selectively 'melt' fat from a specific body area with specific exercises. The only way to lose fat deposits in an offending area is to reduce the overall amount of body fat stored – by cutting calorie intake, exercising aerobically and increasing your muscle mass for example. You can, however, target specific flabby areas that need firming up and tone the muscles beneath fat deposits so they become visible as you lose total body fat.

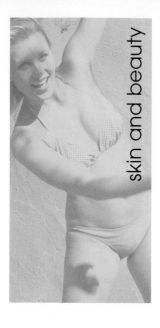

skin and beauty

get beach body ready

Now that you are eating more healthily – for optimum beauty and energy – you are slimmer and more toned, with your skin in good condition, you are getting near to wearing your bikini with confidence. However, before you prepare to bare any flesh make sure that all parts of your body are ready for the beach. Elbows, knees and heels, for example, can be areas of unsightly hard skin that are neglected and for which there are plenty of creams available to improve skin texture.

sun protection for hands

Don't forget your hands when it comes to protecting yourself from the sun's rays. The skin on your hands is very thin and often shows damage, in the form of sun spotting and loss of elasticity, before your face does. Use sunscreen on your hands whenever they will be exposed, even when simply going about everyday activities.

handy hints

Various day-to-day activities take their toll on hands, which are second only to the neck in revealing age. Cold weather, the sun, detergents and too much hot water are all responsible for damaging our skin and weakening fingernails.

If you have dry hands in need of a 'quick-fix', spread plenty of moisturizing cream or petroleum jelly over them. Put on cotton gloves, then snug-fitting latex surgical gloves. Leave the gloves on your hands for at least 2 hours, but preferably overnight. In the morning remove the gloves and you will have beautifully smooth, moisturized hands.

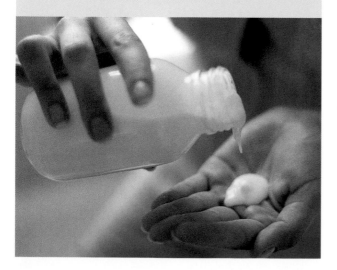

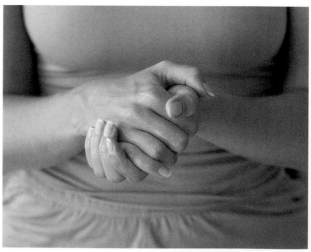

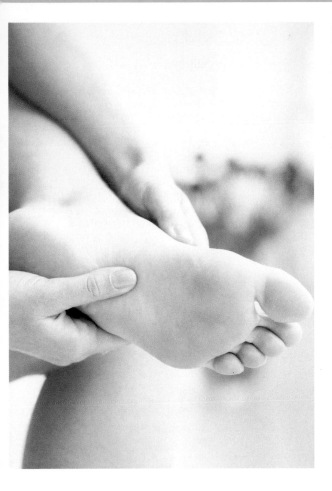

sensible shoe shopping

Remember that shoes that feel tight in the shop will be even worse after a day on your feet. If your feet are different sizes, buy shoes for the larger one.

relaxing treat. It soothes your lower legs and feet and your feet end up with skin like a baby's. Alternatively, give your feet a treat at home by massaging your feet with oil and soaking them in a foot bath.

back to backcare

Just because you canít see your back or reach it easily without a long-handled brush, you cannot afford to ignore it. Like the rest of your body, your back requires some beauty attention, especially if you want to wear a bikini or halter-neck top on holiday.

Beauty salons offer a back 'facial', which involves giving your back some or all of the following: a deep cleansing and exfoliating treatment, steam to relax the pores, extraction of blackheads and blemishes, massage, a treatment mask, toning and moisturizing to leave you feeling hydrated, clean, refreshed and relaxed. Even if you don't have a spotty back your back will benefit from the attention and you will enjoy the pampering experience.

Alternatively, you could treat your back at home with the help of a partner or close friend. First get them to cleanse your back using a facecloth and your normal facial cleanser. Apply an exfoliant (see page 42) then it rinse off. Finally, apply a purifying mask and leave it in place for a while before rinsing this off and finishing with moisturizer if necessary. Even with this do-it-yourself treatment, your back will feel cleaner and tighter.

treat your feet

Our feet deserve more care and attention than they usually receive. They are invariably forgotten until they start to give trouble. On the whole it is neglect and badly fitting shoes rather than any congenital condition that cause problems, and women are four times more likely than men to experience foot problems – high heels are partly to blame.

Your feet are very likely to be on show when you're on a beach holiday – as you go about barefoot or in strappy shoes – so they need to look good. Soften rough, dry feet just as for hands. Apply moisturizer, cover them with cling film to trap your body heat and increase the moisturizer's penetration of the skin, then wear woollen socks over the plastic overnight.

If you can, visit a salon for a pedicure before you go away. A thorough pedicure is a wonderful

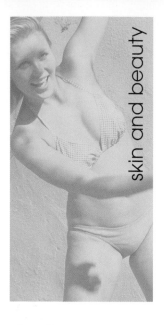

skin and beauty

follicle free

Wearing a bikini means you are exposing more of your body than usual. This fact, combined with the widespread female desire to have smooth hairless skin, means that ensuring underarms, bikini line and legs are hair free is often a priority before going on holiday. There is a huge range of products and techniques currently available for removing unwanted body hair. Of these, shaving is the quickest, easiest and cheapest option.

shaving

Shaving is especially effective for removing hair from legs and underarms. Keeping the skin taut, always shave in the opposite direction of the hair growth. The hair is cut above the surface of the skin so the smooth feel of a close shave is only temporary and regrowth usually occurs within 2–3 days. New regrowth feels coarse because of the angle of the cut but, contrary to popular belief, shaved hair does not grow back thicker.

An electric razor does not give the closest shave but offers the advantage that you will not nick yourself when shaving. It needs to be used on dry skin. With a safety razor, however, you need to wet the area to be shaved thoroughly with warm soapy water. The water hydrates and softens the hair, making it much easier to cut. Rinse and shake excess water off the razor blade rather than wiping it, to preserve the blade's sharpness.

depilatory products

Depilatories – creams, lotions or roll-ons – are painless and easy to apply. The unwanted hair is

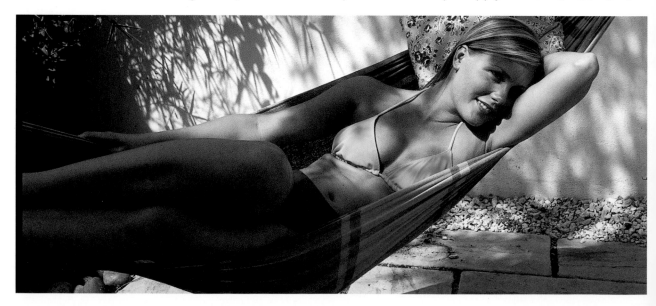

dissolved at the skin's surface and the result lasts longer than if you had shaved. However, the chemicals in depilatories can cause skin irritation, so always test for an adverse reaction by doing a patch test first. To enhance absorption of the depilatory, apply a warm facecloth to the area to soften the hair and open the follicles. Never leave the depilatory on the skin for longer than the recommended time. Wipe it away with a facecloth to help remove more of the hair shaft.

waxing

The best option for the bikini area, waxing results in a clean smooth surface and does not irritate the skin and nerve endings like shaving and depilatory creams do. Waxing is also suitable for legs and thighs but the hair to be removed needs to be at least 5mm (¼in) long for the process to work. The method involces applying hot wax to the skin and pressing a strip of paper or cloth into the wax. The strip is then quickly pulled away, taking the hair with it. Because waxing pulls the hair out below the surface of the skin, the hair grows back finer. You can wax your own legs at home or visit a salon for a half- or full-leg treatment.

underarm shaving

Shaving under your arms reduces the bacteria in the armpits and therefore body odour. Do not apply deodorant or antiperspirant immediately after shaving under your arms – leave it half an hour or so to avoid stinging.

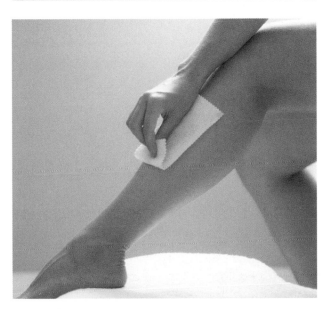

avoiding shaving nicks and rashes

Use a sharp, clean blade (not one that's been lying in water beside the bath!) and don't press too hard as you shave. Do not shave just before exfoliating and don't shave sunburnt skin. Using shaving gel or cream rather than soap for shaving may be kinder to your skin.

A good remedy for skin irritated by shaving is to apply cold, damp camomile tea bags or a cloth soaked in strong cold camomile tea to the affected area.

sugaring

This is a similar method to waxing, which involves applying a warm sugary paste. It tends to be less painful than wax when removed as it does not stick to the skin like wax does.

specialist treatments

Electrolysis is the only truly permanent method of hair removal. A tiny needle is inserted into each hair follicle and zaps the hair down to the root with a short impulse of energy. Each hair is then tweezed out individually. Another semi-permanent option is to remove hair by passing a laser beam through the skin to destroy individual hair follicles. This method works best on light-skinned people with dark hair.

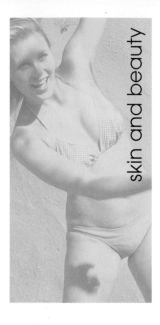

skin and beauty

safe tanning

We tend to look and feel better with a bit of a tan. Attempting to acquire one, however, can be a dangerous business without adequate precautions. The harmful ultraviolet rays in sunlight can cause sunburn and, over time, damage collagen production which ages the skin prematurely. The build-up of damage to the skin can culminate in skin cancer. The safest way of getting that healthy glowing look, therefore, is to get your tan from a bottle.

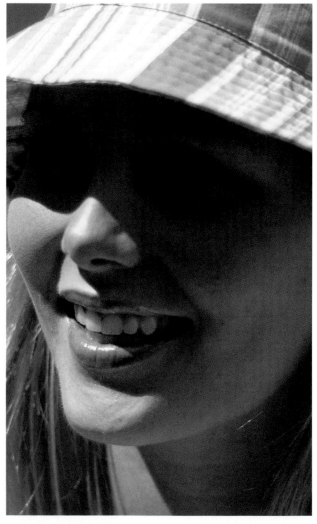

self-tanning

There are plenty of fake tan lotions, 'milks' and sprays on the market, which provide quite a convincing result. Do a patch test first on a hidden place like the soles of your feet. Good skin preparation is necessary for a smooth all-over fake tan – first exfoliate then use a light formula moisturizer all over. Wearing surgical gloves to avoid tell-tale brown palms, apply the self-tan using long, smooth, even strokes and working from your feet up. For a more realistic look on naturally paler areas of skin such as the insides of your arms, mix the tan with a little moisturizer.

sun protection

The skin darkens in response to sunlight or the artificial ultraviolet light of sunbeds. Sun creams containing titanium reflect or completely block ultraviolet light and do not allow tanning. For tanning as well as protection from the sun you need a cream that only partially absorbs ultraviolet light. The degree of protection is expressed as a factor number, known as SPF (sun protection factor). For example, SPF 15 means that you could stay exposed for 15 times longer than the length of time at which your unprotected skin would burn.

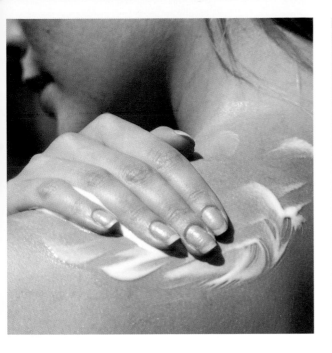

Build up your tan gradually – start with a high factor cream and only an hour in the sun on the first day of your holiday. Burning is not a necessary part of the tanning process and a tan achieved slowly and without burning goes deeper and is therefore likely to last longer. Always use sunscreens that protect against both ultraviolet B (UVB) rays, which cause sunburn, and ultraviolet A (UVA) rays, which cause long-term skin ageing and cancer.

treating sunburn

Sunburn causes long-term damage and is to be avoided at all costs. It is a true burn, with tissue destruction, which happens a few hours after exposure to sun. If you do get sunburnt it may help to take a cool bath or shower or apply cool compresses and take aspirin for the pain. Keep the sunburnt skin moist by regularly applying a non-greasy moisturizing lotion or an after sun product containing ingredients such as aloe vera to cool and rehydrate and vitamins to help the damaged skin. Calamine lotion will help lessen the itching. Consult a doctor for severe sunburn and make sure you stay out of the sun until the skin is completely healed.

sun dos and don'ts

do...
- Cover up or use sunscreen, applying it all over and reapplying it every hour
- Avoid the sun between 11am and 3pm when ultraviolet radiation is greatest
- Wear cotton or silk – they are good barriers
- Ensure your children wear protective clothing, sun hats and sunscreen – the greater their exposure to sun, the higher their risk of skin cancer 20 or more years on
- Protect your eyes as well as your skin. Wear sunglasses that provide 100 per cent UV ray protection
- Stay adequately hydrated
- Be aware that altitude heightens sun damage: the higher you go the more you lose the protective effect of the ozone layer against ultraviolet light.
- Watch your skin and report unusual changes to a doctor

don't...
- Swim without sun protection, thinking water protects your skin – it does not
- Forget to renew your sunscreen after swimming and after every few hours
- Leave your suncare product lying in direct sunlight, nor store it in the fridge
- Neglect to cover all areas with sunscreen – lips, hands and feet are often forgotten
- Have short intensive sunbathing holidays, especially if you are fair-skinned or have more than 100 moles
- Use ultraviolet sunbeds all year long. Excessive use is more damaging to the skin than lying under the hottest sun

picture credits

Corbis UK Ltd/© Anna Palma 74–75 main picture.
Getty Images/Jim Bastardo 6–7 main picture, /Terry Doyle 46–47 main picture, /Peter LaMastro 100–101 main picture.
Octopus Publishing Group Limited/Sandra Lane 20 centre, /Gary Latham 6 centre, 15, 51 top right, 83, 100 centre, 107 top right, 107 bottom right, 107 bottom left, 107 bottom centre, /James Merrell 29 top left, /Peter Myers 51 bottom left, /Peter Pugh-Cook front cover, 2, 4, 5 centre, 7, 8, 9, 12 top left, 12 bottom right, 13, 14 top left, 16 top left, 16 bottom left, 17 top left, 17 top right, 17 bottom right, 17 bottom left, 18 top left, 18 bottom left, 19, 20–21 centre, 22 top left, 22 bottom left, 24 top left, 24 bottom right, 25, 26, 27, 29, 30 top left, 30 centre, 30 bottom right, 31 top centre, 31 top left, 31 centre right, 31 bottom right, 31 bottom centre, 32 left, 32 right, 32 top left, 32 centre, 33 left, 33 right, 33 centre, 34 top left, 34 centre, 35 top left, 35 centre, 35 top right, 35 centre right, 35 bottom right, 36 right, 36 top left, 36 centre, 37 left, 37 right, 37 centre left, 37 centre right, 38 top left, 38 top right, 38 bottom right, 38 bottom left, 39 top left, 39 top right, 39 bottom left, 40 top left, 40 top right, 40 bottom right, 40 bottom left, 41 left, 41 right, 42 top left, 42 bottom right, 42 bottom left, 43 top left, 43 centre right, 43 bottom left, 44 top left, 46–47 centre, 47 centre right, 48 top left, 49, 50 top left, 52 top left, 53, 54 top left, 54 bottom left, 56, 58 top left, 58 bottom right, 59 left, 59 right, 59 centre, 60 top left, 60 centre, 61 left, 61 right, 61 centre, 62 top left, 62 centre, 62 bottom left, 63 top centre, 63 top left, 63 bottom right, 63 bottom left, 64 right, 64 top left, 64 bottom left, 65 top left, 65 bottom right, 65 bottom left, 66 top, 66 centre, 66 bottom, 67 top, 67 centre, 67 bottom, 68 top left, 68 bottom left, 69 left, 69 right, 69 centre left, 69 centre right, 70 top left, 70 bottom left, 71, 72, 73 top left, 73 centre, 73 top right, 73 bottom right, 73 bottom left, 74 centre, 74–75 centre, 75 centre right, 76 top left, 76 bottom left, 78 top left, 80 top left, 80 bottom left, 81, 82 top left, 82 bottom right, 84 right, 84 top left, 84 centre, 85 top centre, 85 top left, 85 bottom right, 85 bottom left, 86 top left, 86 centre, 86 bottom left, 87 top left, 87 top right, 87 bottom right, 87 bottom left, 88 top left, 88 centre, 89 top left, 89 top right, 89 bottom, 90 top left, 90 bottom right, 90 bottom left, 91 top left, 91 top right, 91 bottom right, 91 bottom left, 92 top left, 92 centre left, 92 centre right, 92 bottom right, 93 top left, 93 centre right, 93 bottom left, 94 top, 94 centre, 94 bottom, 95 top, 95 centre, 95 bottom, 96 top left, 96 bottom left, 97 left, 97 right, 97 centre, 98 top centre, 98 top left, 98 top right, 98 bottom left, 98 bottom centre, 99 top centre, 99 top left, 99 top right, 99 bottom left, 100–101 centre, 102 top left, 102 bottom left, 103, 104, 106, 108 right, 108 top left, 108 centre, 109 centre right, 109 bottom left, 109 bottom centre, 110 right, 110 top left, 111 left, 111 right, 111 centre, 112 right, 112 top left, 113 left, 113 right, 113 bottom, 114 top left, 114 bottom right, 114 bottom left, 115 top, 115 centre, 115 bottom, 116 top, 116 centre, 117 top, 117 centre, 117 bottom, 118 top, 118 centre, 118 bottom, 119 top, 119 centre, 120 top left, 120 bottom right, 120 bottom left, 122 top left, 122 bottom, 123, 124 top left, 124 bottom left, 125, /William Reavell 5 top, 5 bottom, 14 bottom left, 23, 28 left, 28 right, 46 centre, 52 bottom left, 57 bottom left, 77, 78 centre left, 79, /Simon Smith 50 bottom left, 57 top right, 105 top left, 105 bottom right, /Ian Wallace 21 centre right, 44 bottom right, 45 left, 45 right, 55, 101 right, 121, /Mark Winwood 48 bottom left.
Image State 20–21 main picture.

acknowledgements

Executive Editor Doreen Palamartschuk-Gillon
Managing Editor Clare Churly
Editor Jo Lethaby
Executive Art Editor Joanna Bennett
Designer Geoff Borin
Special Photography Peter Pugh-Cook
Picture Research Zoë Holtermann
Production Controller Lucy Woodhead

The publisher wishes to thank Marks & Spencer for the loan of bikinis for the book.

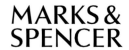

**MARKS &
SPENCER**